WHEN THE NIGHTINGALE SANG

A Nurse's Life in the 1950s and 1960s

As told to:

Rosalind Franklin

Meadow Books, Burgess Hill

First Published in the United Kingdom by:

Meadow Books

35, Stonefield Way, Burgess Hill, West Sussex, RH15 8DW

Tel: (01444) 239044

Email: MeadowBooks@hotmail.com

Website: www.stores.ebay.co.uk/meadowbooks

1st Edition, November 2004

ISBN 0-9515655-3-2

Text Design by Rosalind Franklin

Cover Design by Larry Smith: email blsmith@comcast.net

Introduction

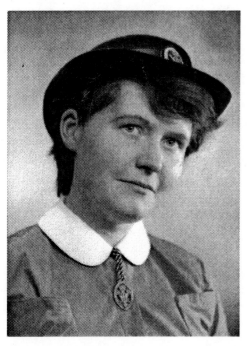

Cynthia O'Neill nee Carstairs (SRN, SCM, QN, HV) (pictured left in 1964) started her SRN training in 1956 at Hammersmith Hospital, London, a time when the NHS was at its peak, and a nurse was not expected to speak unless spoken to. After qualifying in 1959, Cynthia went on to do part I of her Midwifery training at Queen Charlottes Hospital, and part II at Thorpe Coombe in the East End of London.

After further Queen's Nurse and Health Visitor training in London, Cynthia went to work as a Queen's District Nursing Sister, Midwife and School Nurse in East Sussex in 1961.

Cynthia O'Neill is now retired from nursing, and writes and lectures on nursing history. She has written two other books: *'A Picture of Health; Hospitals and Nursing on old Picture Postcards'* (ISBN 0-9515655-0-8) and *'More Pictures of Health'* (ISBN 0-9515655-1-6), both available from Meadow Books. (Order details on the back page)

Rosalind Franklin is a freelance writer who lives in the West Country.

Note

This is my true story. However, I have changed most of the names of members of staff and patients out of respect.

If the names of the people in this book bear any similarity with the name of a person, either living or dead, it is entirely coincidental, and nothing should be taken or implied from it.

Cynthia O'Neill

Burgess Hill, November 2004

"Lectured at by Committees, preached at by chaplains, scowled on by treasurers and stewards, scolded by matrons, sworn at by surgeons, bullied by dressers, grumbled at and abused by patients, insulted if old and ill-favoured, talked flippantly to if middle-aged and good humoured, seduced if young – they are what any woman would be under the same circumstances."

L Clendening

INDEX

CHAPTER I	I bet you won't stick it	11
CHAPTER II	It's not all fluffing up pillows	21
CHAPTER III	You will only speak when spoken to	30
CHAPTER IV	Onwards and Upwards	41
CHAPTER V	The World holds its breath	56
CHAPTER VI	Oh, come all ye faithful	68
CHAPTER VII	A Long Hard Night	74
CHAPTER VIII	Getting a Set of Wheels	88
CHAPTER IX	Grey Becomes Blue	99
CHAPTER X	Crash, Bang, Wallop!	112
CHAPTER XI	Stork Duty	128
CHAPTER XII	A Pregnant Pause	140
CHAPTER XIII	A Royal Duty	151
CHAPTER XIV	Salad Days	159
CHAPTER XV	Sussex Ups and Downs	166
CHAPTER XVI	Don't forget to put the Kettle on	179

CHAPTER I
'I Bet You Won't Stick At It'

June 25th 1956 was one of those hot sultry summer days. The sky was a brilliant shade of blue, and quoting one of my mother's favourite sayings, there weren't enough white patches in the sky for even a skilful tailor to make a shirt with.

'I'm off to become a nurse today,' I whispered to Ginger, my family's four-year-old Tomcat, 'I'll miss you, but be a good boy, won't you?' I kissed his soft fur affectionately.

Today was the day I'd been waiting for, impatiently counting off the days, hours and minutes until its arrival, on a Borough's adding machine at work in my boring office job. I'd been working in the accounts office at the large local bakery, J Lyons and Co. Ltd, since leaving school at the age of seventeen and a quarter, and was only biding my time there until I had reached eighteen, and was deemed old enough to begin nurses' training.

Now, finally, the big day had arrived. In just a little while, I'd be starting the nursing adventure that would last me a lifetime. I spent the final moments of that hot June morning in the small garden of the large grey, once red-bricked, rented Victorian terraced town house, that was my family home and the house in which my mother had been born in in 1908.

Such an old house reverberated with many memories. Mum laughed as she told us the story of her younger brother, Terry, having his tonsils taken out on the oak kitchen table in 1912. I sat listening to Mum's stories, wide-eyed with my five younger brothers and sisters, and always wanted to cry when Mum listed the many family friends who had frequently visited our home, but never returned after being sent to the bloody French battlefields of World War 1.

Now it was *my* turn to leave the house, and make a step into the unknown for a life of dedication and sacrifice in my nursing vocation. And I was under no illusion that I would have to sacrifice much in order to live a nurse's life. But nursing was something I *had* to do, whatever the cost.

I had always wanted to be a nurse. Growing up as the eldest girl in a family of six children, putting the needs of others first had been required of me since I'd been a young age. At convent school, it had been instilled into me to have mercy, and to sacrifice my needs to care for others. This was one of the few worthwhile things, I felt, that the nuns had taught me.

I had been bored senseless in most of my school lessons, the nuns trying their best to keep my attention during endless French Vocabulary drills and Shakespearean Sonnets. My one aim had been to leave the local Convent of the Sacred Heart in Hammersmith, London, with, at the very least, the minimum qualifications necessary to enter Student Nurse training. I did, obtaining four 'O' levels.

I realised later, that the essential qualifications for a nurse were less easy to assess at the beginning of her training. Courage, determination, a stomach of iron and a very strong back, a love of one's neighbour regardless of class, colour or creed, and a certain amount of humility were all vital.

In realising my nursing goal, I had tried to prepare myself as best I could during my teenage years. When I was fourteen, I'd replied to a recruitment advertisement from the Ministry of Labour and National Service that I'd seen in one of Mum's woman's magazines. As fifteen was a common age for school-leavers to go into their various trades and apprenticeships, I hoped that I'd be able to start nurse training the following year.

I was bitterly disappointed, however, when the Ministry informed me that I'd have to wait until I was 18 to train. However, they encouraged me to prepare myself in the meantime, by getting as much first aid training under my belt before then. As well as doing as much First-Aid as possible in the Girl Guides, I'd joined the local St. John Ambulance Brigade Cadets.

Every Monday evening after school, I went along with my best friend Anne to a cold church basement at the end of King Street. There, the Cadet Officers taught me many skills such as bandaging, taking temperatures, simple home nursing and first aid. St John's standards were extremely high, and the early discipline instilled in me proved invaluable.

Sister Ilfa Jones, a theatre sister from Charring Cross Hospital, helped train us cadets. She gave Anne and I great encouragement to become fully trained nurses, warning us, however, that nursing was not for the faint-hearted and was very hard work.

Meanwhile, our Hammersmith SJAB entered a team into the 1954 District First Aid competition and won the Silver Challenge Cup, much to the delight of our cadet officers, Mrs Donne and Miss Naismith.

As SJAB cadets, we were required to do voluntary work, and apart from doing shopping and gardening for old folks on Saturday afternoons, I was able to extend my voluntary duties to help out at Hammersmith Hospital when I had reached seventeen years of age.

Young and eager, I reported for my first sample of hospital life, quite unprepared for all the foul smells and frightening sounds expelling from the sick and dying. On my first day on a ward, I was terrified. Still drowsy or unconscious patients returned from theatre with bulky black rubber airways attached to their mouths, and strong smells of anaesthetic gas expired from these airways filling the ward. The gas along with the stench of urine, vomit and cleaning materials made the ward's aura all rather over-whelming.

However, despite wanting to gag, I persevered, and assisted on the hospital wards every week for a year. On 6.30pm each Tuesday evening, wearing a starched white apron over my grey cotton SJAB cadet uniform dress, and a stiff white butterfly-type cap to keep my hair tidy, I was let loose. For two hours, I helped out as best as I could on ward C6, one of the female surgical wards of the large seven-hundred bed hospital. I was perhaps more of a nuisance than a help, but I tried my best, and looked forward to my weekly sessions there.

My first task on Tuesday evenings was usually to help a nurse wash a patient after an operation. It was important that all patients recovering from surgery were out of their operating gowns, and washed and freshly groomed, ready for any visitors that they might have later that evening.

I then went from bed to bed, collecting the kidney dishes filled with post-operative vomit.* The dishes were taken to the sluice where they were emptied, cleaned, and sterilised, ready for their next outing.

Visiting time on each ward was between 7.15pm and 7.45pm and had a strict set of rules. There were never, *ever* exceptions to the visiting rules. Two visiting cards per patient were allowed, and *only* two visitors at any one time were allowed at the bedside. Children were never allowed to visit. A nurse meticulously policed visits from the ward entrance, carefully filling a shiny stainless steel trolley with the collected visiting cards.

I flitted around the ward, ensuring each bed had enough wooden chairs for visitors to sit on. Flowers brought in by the visitors were then carefully trimmed and arranged in vases, to be later whisked out of the ward to keep their lonely all-night vigil in the corridors. It was said by Matron, that these cheerful companions to otherwise sterile and austere surroundings gobbled up the oxygen in the wards at night.

---

* In 1955, sickness was common after anaesthetic, and the patient was subject to far more post-operative complications than nowadays. There was also a far longer recovery period. A patient would *never* be released the same day after having a general anaesthetic.

At 7.45pm the ward bell tinkled as the notorious, 'Time to go, please Visitors!' echoed around the ward. As crowds dutifully milled out through the doors, Sister, easily identified by her navy dress and frilly lace-trimmed cap of honour, answered the questions plied to her by anxious relatives, in her overly polished office overlooking the ward.

I had unfortunately not been around on the day when a very important visitor came to visit Hammersmith Hospital. On 6th June 1955, Queen Elizabeth II was escorted around the wards to meet some of the patients. The hospital was buzzing for many days after the visit. The patients' and staff's experiences echoed around the wards.

'Did you see her? She's even more beautiful in the flesh...'

'She asked how I was feeling. God bless her! Her kind words have done me the power of good.'

'She came and shook my hand and said, 'How do you do?''

They weren't all positive memories of the Queen's visit though. One of the junior nurses on C6 muttered to me that she was stuck scrubbing soiled bed sheets in the sluice at the time of the Queen's visit.

'The patients don't stop crapping the bed for the Queen!' Mary grumbled.

'I was stuck doing French at school!' I said.

'Poor you!' Mary pulled a face. 'Never mind! Come on, Carstairs, it's time to do the dressing's drums.'

After the visitors left on a Tuesday evening, heavy stainless steel drums, used for packing dressings, were cleaned with ether meth., and then polished up to a shine. The drums were then repacked with the cotton wool balls, facemasks and the gauze dressings ready for the hospital porter to collect later that evening to take to be 'autoclaved' (steam sterilised). Some of the cotton wool balls that were repacked into the drum looked as weary as the sleepy night nurse who had rolled them the night before. It would be my last duty before 'knocking off' at night to ensure that these drums were clearly labelled 'C6', so that they found their way back to the correct ward.

The number 72 bus to and from the hospital was notoriously infrequent, and I often arrived home very late after one of my voluntary shifts. However, this and the ghastly sights, smells and rushed routine were not enough to sway me from my resolve to be a nurse. My SJAB voluntary experience did nothing to deter me from coming back for more; a glutton for punishment, I had even applied to train at the very same hospital where I volunteered, Hammersmith Hospital.

I was accepted after a gruelling interview with the silver-haired Matron Godden, and duly prepared for my big day.

The first stage of the three-year State Registered Nurse (SRN) training was a three-month course called a Preliminary Training School (PTS). Being resident in the nurse's home or 'living-in' as it was referred to, was compulsory for the first six months of training, no matter how close one lived to the hospital.

Despite the fact that Hammersmith Hospital was only seven miles down the road from my family home, it was therefore compulsory that I 'live-in' at their Nurses Home, Hammersmith House, for a time.

My pale-green trunk, that had cost me a princely £10, was packed ready with the items that had been on the *'list of items required by students entering nurse's training school'* sent by Matron, together with a few other bits and bobs. I had scrimped and saved very hard for these items. The items on the list totalled £25, and money did just not grow on trees for my working class family.

List of items required by Students Entering Nurses' Training School

Birth Certificate

National Insurance card

P45

£2.10 shillings for books

Ruler, pen, pencils (some coloured) and rubber

Scissors

Watch with second hand if possible or pulse meter

White blouse and black shorts for physical training

Gym shoes or tennis shoes

Grey stockings (artificial silk or heavyweight nylon)

Plain black shoes with laces, moderate heels, with rubbers - two pairs if possible. A suitable variety of 'duty shoe' can be obtained from Daniel Neal of Kensington High Street.

If it is desired to wear outdoor uniform, a navy blue gabardine coat and navy hat or storm cap should be provided.

My mother was unfortunately unable to help me financially. I was the eldest of six children in a one-parent family, my father, an alcoholic, having been sent packing from the home. My brothers and sisters were all still at school, Diana at 16 had just sat her 'O' levels, John at 15 was working hard hoping to study engineering with the Royal Navy, and Lucille, 14, Frank, 12 and Madeleine aged 10 were yet undecided.

My weekly wage from my Lyons office job was £4, 10 shillings. After tax and National Insurance, and paying Mum for my keep, I was left with about £2 a week. It took a lot of pay packets to save up for nursing training, and I worked a lot of overtime so I could afford all the items on

Matron Godden's list.

The necessary watch with a second hand was an expensive and luxury item in 1956. My Timex watch cost £2, 12 shillings and sixpence; over a week's take-home pay. The black leather-soled laced duty shoes came from Daniel Neal of Kensington High Street and cost £3, 6 shillings and three pence, a pair...and I needed two pairs.

To be different, or let's say awkward, the School demanded grey stockings, which were much more expensive and harder to obtain than the traditional black nurse's hose, but they insisted on grey, so grey it had to be. I bought six pairs of Pretty Polly grey fishnet stockings at 6/11 a pair. Instead of laddering, these went into small holes and then went into bigger holes with all the bending and stretching we did. These were held up with 'roll-ons' with suspenders attached.

Compulsory P.E. was forced on all nursing students, so a new white Aertex shirt costing £2, 2 shillings, and my old school shorts, plimsolls and socks had been carefully placed in my green trunk. Although I loved playing hockey and tennis, I didn't like the sound of enforced group P.E. one little bit!

My mother gave me a Bible and pretty red travel clock, and these were packed along with two pairs of new cornflower blue pyjamas into my green trunk. *

Lyons Bakery were sorry to see me leave, and tried to tempt me to stay by offering me a lucrative well-paid job with lots of perks, teaching staff in their Training School. The J. Lyons factory employed 30,000 people at its peak, so there was plenty of room for career expansion, even for a young woman like me in the un-liberated 1950s. Lyons assured me this job opening

---

* I grew to love this faithful little red alarm clock; ringing out at some very odd hours, it lasted me for over 25 years.

would still be open, if I ever decided that the long hours, petty discipline, hard work and lack of free time involved with nursing training was not to my liking.

My pale green trunk had been packed, checked, and rechecked. I was inpatient now. I sat in my mother's heavily scented back garden, excited and scared all at the same time. Now and again, a blackbird or sparrow hopped down from the wall, taking the food scraps left out for them when they thought Ginger or I weren't looking. The perfume from the carefully tended roses was heady, only adding to my sense of anticipation. I breathed in the scent and sighed deeply.

I particularly loved the scent and colour of the 'Madame Butterfly' rose with its delicate pale peach petals. Now I was waving goodbye to my favourite Puccini diva, and 'George Dickson' and 'Lady Sylvia' too, for Nurses' Preliminary Training School at Hammersmith Hospital, and crossed my fingers that Mum would care for these beautiful roses well in my absence. Mum came out into the garden to say goodbye to me. She was all dressed up 'to the nines' for a day's work as an extra at the Elstree film studios.

Mum had worked with many stars and starlets, and today she was working with Bob Monkhouse. Mum didn't think much of Bob Monkhouse, she thought he was far too crude, but she only had good things to say about Stewart Granger. 'Now he's a gentleman,' she said. She had modelled for a painting used in the film 'Footsteps in the Fog' that he'd been the lead star in, and this set prop now took pride of place above the fireplace in our family's living room.

'I'm sorry that I can't see you off properly. I have to go now, but I'm so proud of you, Cynth.' Mum said, tears whelming up in her eyes.

I know Hammersmith Hospital was only seven miles down the road, but it was going to be a big wrench to be parted from my close-knit family. I spent the last half hour nervously checking and rechecking my appearance in the hall mirror, as I paced up and down waiting for my taxi. Ginger meowed as he wound his soft body around my legs, looking affectionately up at me. As he purred contentedly, he seemed to say,

'The best of British luck to you, for your training, Cynthia, but I bet you won't stick it!'

Indeed, in the past few weeks my head had been filled with disturbing tales of nurses being bullied and ill-treated. I wondered if I *would* stick it. My best friend, Anne, as she was a few months older than me, had already started training at Hammersmith. Despite her horror stories, I had been so jealous of her, but now my time had finally come!

The taxi pulled up at 2.30pm, as booked. The taxi driver, Bob, who was a neighbour, had known me since I was a little girl in pigtails. He, like Mum, looked slightly whimsical.

'Gordon Bennett, Cynth., anyone was thinking you're going to Africa or sommat, not just down the road!' Bob complained, struggling to lift my heavy, tightly packed trunk into the taxi.

The taxi pulled off, and as I leant back into Bob's black leather seats, I thought,

'I'm finally leaving my childhood behind.'

From a radio nearby, that week's Number One chart single 'I'll Be Home' by Pat Boone was playing. I would be home someday, but today I was too busy looking *forward* to glance back at my house; too excited by what lay ahead. My mouth felt dry, my heart raced, and I felt butterflies in my stomach.

CHAPTER II
'It's Not All Fluffing Up Pillows'

Hammersmith Hospital, formerly the Hammersmith Workhouse, was rather a stark looking redbrick building with a green clock tower. There were no pretty fountains or greenery to greet an arrival, just plain unadulterated brickwork.

A friendly-looking man in a smart dark-green uniform with peaked cap waved Bob's cab through the gate. Seeing the pale-faced nervous looking teenager with her smartest dress on, he immediately guessed the cab's destination. With a nod and broad smile, Mr James, The Head Porter on the Gate, directed us to the Nurse's Home.

I'd made sure that I had not spent my last fifteen shillings, taken from my post office savings book just the day before, so that I had enough money to pay my taxi fare. As I fumbled to get my purse out, Bob refused to take my fare. I wondered if he knew that if he had taken my money, I would have had nothing left until payday.

'Thank you, Mr Townsend.' I blushed.

'No problem, just remember me, if me or the Missus is ever on one of your wards. Gawd help us!' and chuckling to himself, Bob reset the taxi meter and drove off.

I stood gazing at the Nurse's Home, 'Hammersmith House,' which although greying was sparkling in today's brilliant sunshine. The building was dotted with numerous bedroom windows, and I wondered which would be mine as I straightened my dress, and nervously smoothed down my hair for the umpteenth time. An impatient cough coming from one of the stern looking women standing at the doors interrupted my thoughts, and I obediently hurried up the meticulously scrubbed steps.

The Nurses' Home Sister, a plump, elderly, grey-haired woman, and some of the other PTS Sister Tutors stood waiting for their new arrivals or 'inmates'. The assembled group greeted me with a formal handshake, and a cold smile, ticking my name off their long list of names. The Sisters' manner was rather militaristic, and there was little warmth in their welcome. I was so scared that I immediately scuttled to their commands without asking anything. This was just the way the Sisters wanted to keep it.

Home Sister handed me my room key, and my first job was to find my room and unpack. I heaved my trunk up and down through the Nurse's Home corridors, passing lots of other girls doing the exact same thing, searching for their own rooms, until I found my room, number 207.

The small room allotted to me as my bedroom rather resembled a hospital side ward. The walls were tatty and peeling, and the plain furniture was designed for practicality rather than beauty.

There was a dark wooden wardrobe, dressing table, desk and uncomfortable wicker chair, and there was a small sink in the corner with white bakelite tooth mug perched by its side. A ragged brown rug covered part of the polished wooden floor. Covering the old iron framed bed was a pale green bedspread exactly of the type used on the hospital's wards.

On top of the bed, my PTS uniform was laid out ready, let out or taken in as per my list of measurements sent to Matron Godden some weeks before. An old family friend and neighbour, Cicely, had helped measure me, so that the exact length of my dress off the ground was 12 inches. Even for the 1950's this was considered to be a rather long dress, but these were the days when male patients were not allowed any glimpse of what they shouldn't see when nurse bent over!

My name had already been written for me on each uniform item laid out on the bed. The starched white dresses and caps had been patched, darned, and re-darned, and the many names of the dresses' users before me had been blackened over with marker pen. The nurse's uniform had been patched so frequently, anyone would have thought cloth rationing was still in place.

Of course, I had to try my dress on before doing anything else. I gazed back at the reflection staring at me from the small mirror over the enamel sink. Once stripped of all make-up, nail polish and jewellery, the office clerk was suddenly transformed into a student nurse. I'd been in a dream-like state all day, and now suddenly, everything seemed very real to me, and was staring out at me from the mirror. The all-white dress was a symbol of purity of mind and body of the student entering the nursing profession, and I felt rather like a novice nun.

My room was stark and bare, but any thought of making it feel more homely was shattered. There was a notice pinned firmly on the wall, reminding all student nurses that no items or pictures could be put on the walls. It also instructed that bedroom slippers must not be kept on the floor. My much loved pictures of home, Ginger and the 18th Hammersmith Girl Guide's Company that I had been so much part of, and had just gained my Lieutenant's Warrant from, would have to stay in my drawer.

I looked out of my window to see what my view was like. I could not believe it; I was overlooking the 'Scrubbs'! The dirty old grey imposing sight of Her Majesty's Prison, Wormwood Scrubbs, and the dismal sight of its barred windows, greeted me each morning, and I was not the only nurse who would be shocked over the next few months to see prisoners peering from across the way into my window, and waving or jeering as they did so. Coincidentally, Wormwood Scrubbs housed seven hundred inmates, the same number of beds as were at the hospital.

After finishing unpacking my things, I made my way for the new PTS's welcome tea in the Nurse's Home. Each table was neatly covered with a white cotton tablecloth, on which a plate of sliced brown and white bread sat. One slice of bread, one pat of butter, and one small cake or Lyon's Jam tart were allocated per trainee. This made up the 'tea' together with as much tea as we could drink.

The fresh PTS group of nervous teenagers chattered over hospital issue teacups and saucers, and friendships started on that afternoon, some of which were to last for many years. Forty-seven girls as excited and apprehensive as I started on the June 1956 set. My PTS was an international group, with three Irish, two Welsh, and two German girls, and a Canadian, Nigerian, Indian, and a Maltese girl. The Irish girls came to train in England, as they had to pay for their nurse's training back home in Ireland.

'This will be a good craick, eh girls?' said Teresa from County Clare, attempting to break the ice amongst the more reserved English girls.

At my table, sat three English girls; Shirley, Claire and Trudy. Shirley, Claire and I couldn't help but notice the beautiful engagement ring hung on a gold chain around Trudy's neck, and soon a group of girls were crowded around Trudy wanting to hear all about her fiancé.

'What does he do?' asked Claire.

'Is he dishy?' I asked.

'Does he drive?' asked Shirley.

Trudy's fiancé sounded very nice, and we were all very impressed that he drove an Austin Healey Sprite. Most guys we knew didn't have a car, let alone own an Austin Healey Sprite.

'He's a medical student!' Trudy confided in us.

'Oooh!' we all giggled. I warmed to the other girls, particularly Shirley, right away, and we soon became firm friends.

After tea, we were marched off to have a chest x-ray and medical exam, despite all of us already having been passed as fit and healthy by our own GPs, who had filled out complicated lengthy medical questionnaires on our behalf.

'What a waste of time!' I thought.

Sister Tutor Smythe-Jones acted as chaperone during the exam. She seemed to take great delight in leering at me, stripped to my panties. It made me feel very uncomfortable. *

'She's a lesbian!' I overheard a couple of the other girls whisper, but I didn't know what a lesbian was, and was too afraid to ask.

Later that same evening, we were led up to be interviewed, one by one, by Miss Smythe-Jones. Once again, we were required to give our reasons for wanting to be nurses. While waiting our turn in line, we each had to copy 'The Florence Nightingale Pledge for Nurses' into our notebooks. I imagined the hundreds of other nurses from numerous other Preliminary Training School sets who had passed in a similar line before me, writing the very same thing as I.

The Florence Nightingale Pledge for Nurses

'I solemnly pledge myself before God and in the presence of this assembly, to pass my life in purity and to practice my profession faithfully. I will abstain from whatever is deleterious and mischievous, and will not take or knowingly administer any harmful drug. I will do all in my power to maintain and elevate the standard of my profession, and will hold in confidence all personal matters committed to my keeping and all family affairs coming to my knowledge in the practice of my calling. With loyalty will I endeavour to aid the physician in his work, and devote myself to the welfare of those committed to my care.'

---

* The medical failed to find the Scoliosis in my back that would later cause me a great deal of trouble, but I'm inclined to think that Hammersmith were so short of nurses, they grabbed all they could from home and abroad. Had I known of my back problem, I would have still persisted with my training anyway. I was an infatuated teenager, in love with the idea of nursing.

On the inner cover, in each of our notebooks, we were also instructed to inscribe 'The International Code of Ethics for Nurses'. After being given the third degree from Miss Smythe-Jones, I was abruptly dismissed;

'Matron will talk to you all tomorrow. You need to be here for 8am sharp and I do not want to see you wearing any jewellery, even earrings. I do not tolerate any make-up or nail polish, and your hair must be tidy and off the collar. Do not forget your Kirby grips and caps. Supper is at seven. You may go.'

After a leisurely supper with lots more 'getting to know you' chatter, I made my way back to room 207 with its bleak view. Although I hated the view, I realised I would have little time to look out of the window anyway. After double-checking that my little red alarm clock was set at the correct time, I made an early night of it, and although excited, slept soundly in the creaking iron-framed bed.

~ ~ ~ ~ ~ ~ ~ ~ ~ ~ ~ ~

Our PTS School was a small building attached to the Nurse's Home. On entering the School to the right, was a large bright Practical room complete with hospital beds, glistening stainless steel trolleys, red rubber tubes, sterilisers, face-mask jars and shining instrument cupboards full of a variety of obnoxious looking items. The room had a distinct smell of Brasso, Windolene, Carbolic Solution, Vim, Lysol and other polishes blended together with the NHS issue furniture.

Mrs Smith, the room's model patient lived in that room. Mrs Smith was a dummy made in 1950 and could not speak, vomit, or mess the bed. A student nurse could pass a Ryle's tube or a rectal tube right up her and she never complained. Dear Mrs Smith!

Next to the practical room sat the office of Principal PTS tutor, Miss Smythe-Jones, and next to her office were three toilets kept spotlessly clean by us students. Further to the right, was a rather gloomy looking classroom.

The dark grey prison opposite blotted out most of its light, and the highly placed windows were specially designed to stop us gazing out of them during lessons anyway.

Desks and chairs were lined up in strict military fashion. Although students, we were expected to dress in itchy starched white dresses that were as stiff as boards, with our heads adorned with silly white hats. Sitting in this garb on hard over-polished chairs, was not particularly conducive to our learning.

Our lectures were 'talk and chalk', using a large blackboard. A life-size fully coloured plastic model of a male human being, showing his anatomy from head to groin was placed to the left of the blackboard. He didn't have any arms or legs, and of course, his private parts were missing! However, he was very lifelike. I hated him, and he gave me horrible nightmares.

To the opposite side of the room, suspended from a chain from the ceiling, hung Jimmy the 'Skelly'. He was a real skeleton. I wondered who his 'owner' had been and if he had ever realised what his bones were going to be used for after his death. We all grew to quite like Jimmy though, as he was harmless and never rude or insulting to us, unlike most of the tutors who took a peculiar delight in making us feel like the lowest of the low and more than stupid.

I soon learned the daily drill-routine. Quite lengthy prayers commenced each day and were compulsory. Led by Principal Sister Tutor, Miss Smythe-Jones, they lasted fifteen minutes. As a practising Roman Catholic, I asked on the first day to be excused from these prayers as they were conducted in a Protestant manner. It was my right to do this, and as a young girl not long out of convent school, with all its indoctrination, it was what I had been brought up to do. Miss Smythe-Jones turned pale with rage and answered,

27

'Nurse Carstairs! You have come here to be a nurse, and your religion has nothing to do with it.' Her hat bobbled on her head as she shook with anger. I had committed the mortal sin by speaking before being spoken to, and not only that, I was also daring to 'question the system'. Miss Smythe-Jones' tone of voice was very intimidating, but I could not see what I had done wrong.

I'm certain I scored a 'black mark' in my copybook early on because of my request. However, Miss Smythe-Jones had to agree to it. I'd never been spoken to so rudely before, but I bit my lip, determined to put up with this nasty woman as best as I could. This resolve was to prove very difficult and Miss Smythe-Jones made the Lyons' job offer became ever more appealing over the coming months.

Instead of 'Probationers' we were called student nurses, but in no way were we akin to normal students because of the long hours and type of work we did. It was a very long day, and many of us were more than surprised to learn that it was also our duty to thoroughly clean the PTS daily, including all the toilets and the windows.

We were to be in PTS for 8am sharp, and every morning we had to do twenty minutes cleaning duties after prayers. Every nook, cranny and surface was to be made spotless by us so-called 'students.'

There was a rotation chart of duties for us to do, so there was no escaping the more unpleasant jobs such as cleaning the loos, or the more silly jobs such as cleaning the already clean inkwells and pen nibs. The duties also included dusting and polishing furniture, sorting out dirty linen, folding and arranging sheets in a cupboard to military precision, and cleaning the windows. Everything had to be exactly 'so'.

Watched over by all four of the tutors that first morning, our every movement was noted and criticised. Cries came from all over the building of, 'Oh, Nurse, that is not the way to do it', 'Move the table back to the *exact* position you found it, Nurse', 'The pen nibs are still dirty', and 'Really Nurse, you must put the brush right *around* the lavatory pan'. This was all supposed to be part of the toughening up process to be a nurse.

At 8.40am, we all had to squash over one bucket to wash our dusters and then hung them out to dry on the line. All day long, forty-seven yellow dusters danced on the PTS washing line drying. At 8.45am, standing in a line with our hands behind backs, our work was inspected by the unsmiling tutors, and we then had to ask permission to be excused, to which came the sharp response,

'Have you done your job properly?'

Woe betides anyone who had failed in her duty! One young nurse from Berkshire decided her vocation was not in cleaning the toilets and told her tutor in no uncertain manner what she thought of it all. She left the PTS that same morning, followed half an hour later by a girl from Hackney.

After our nervous affirmations that we'd done our tasks correctly, we were dismissed to go and make our beds. Home Sister would have already checked each of our rooms to see that our beds had been stripped to air. Up until just a few years before our school, this few minutes would also have been the time used for our nurse predecessors to change into their clean aprons.

Matron Godden, OBE, a lady of generous proportions, with almost white hair, officially opened the school later that morning with her customary pep talk. Peering over her gold-rimmed glasses, she told us that we had chosen a very hard calling that would not only entail 'fluffing up pillows'. I had already seen that this statement was no exaggeration, as it was only a few hours into the PTS and two students had already walked out.

CHAPTER III
'You Will Only Speak When Spoken To'

Hammersmith Hospital was originally a workhouse, and as far as all of us PTS students were concerned, it was *still* a workhouse. In out time there, we would become regimented, set to military timing, and conditioned to obey orders without questioning. We were here to learn, and our first lesson was to never speak without being spoken to, and to assume we were nitwits and knew nothing.

Lectures started at 9am and went on until 5.30pm. The first lecture we received on our PTS was on the 'Hammersmith High Cap'. We were introduced to the art of making this cap from a piece of cloth board. Perched high on the head, and kept in place by white Kirby grips, this hat was supposed to prevent fleas from a patient hopping onto the nurse's hair, but in practice, the fleas were very persistent and would find a way.

The starch in my dress was rubbing against my neck and the polished chairs were very slippery. It was hard to keep still as Matron preached. She went on a bit.

The tutors doled out the textbooks and hardbound writing books necessary for my course, at the same time extracting the money to pay for these items from me. A timetable was then given out along with a stern reminder to *never* be late for anything.

With the first lecture over, we had a coffee break of half an hour. This enabled us to get to the staff restaurant for nice freshly brewed coffee and rich tea biscuits. The restaurant was a fair walk over the quadrant from the school, and there was always a queue, so we needed this time to get us all fed and watered.

Full board and lodging was provided as part of my training package, and I was given a small monthly training allowance of about £8 which was subject to tax and National Insurance deductions. Shoes and stockings had to be paid for, as well as stationary and other bits and bobs out of this. Nurse's scissors had a habit of going on walkabout and these had to be regularly repurchased at 8 shillings and 6 pence a pair.

After coffee break came another pep talk from Miss Smythe-Jones,

'Men friends are *never* allowed in the bedrooms. There is a small room by the front door where you can meet.'

What a cold unpleasant room this 'nookie' room was, with two hard-backed chairs set primly apart. Romance was never in the air in these formal surroundings!

The list of school rules continued.

'You will only speak when spoken to. You will never run, unless for a fire or haemorrhage. Should you feel ill you will report to myself, and then I will send you to Home Sister, but remember…' Miss Smythe-Jones pursed her lips as she stressed her words, '…you are here to nurse and not to be nursed. Any time off sick of more than three weeks will cause you to do an extra three months training.' The scowling look on Miss Smythe-Jones's face, and her tone of voice showed she meant business. It was an early warning to us all to *never* approach the sick bay.

Once we got on the wards, we soon learned that when we were unwell, the first hurdle was to get past the Ward Sister. She would take our temperatures, asking in a sarcastic voice how we felt. Once we'd got past her, it was far easier; up in 'Sick Clinic' Dr. Wimbush, or 'Daddy Wimbush' as he was christened by his adoring nurse fans, could not have been kinder to us.

'It's all a bit strict, isn't it?' whispered Sheila from her desk next to me, 'I thought I'd joined the *Health* Service, not *National* Service!'

On three mornings a week after coffee break, we filed to the practical room to receive demonstrations on the art of bed making, applying dressings, and getting the patient out of bed. Mrs Smith would receive the best personal care and attention from forty five anxious student nurses. Turned from side to side, her sheets were changed and she was made as comfortable as a dummy can be.

The other two weekday mornings were spent being put through 'physical jerks'. The roll call was made to ensure no nurse could escape. We did not question why we had to do PE. Outside in the yard next to the premature Baby unit, but overlooked by B Block, our antics in our white shirts and black shorts ensured that patients looking out from nearby ward windows got free entertainment.

Lunch and supper was taken in the staff restaurant with a choice of menu offered to waitress service. Tables were always laid neatly with starched white cotton tablecloths, shining cutlery and water jugs and menu cards. Following the trek there and back and having to queue in a long line, meant little time to actually eat, and meals proved to be rushed affairs. We student nurses became, by necessity, champions of gobbling with gusto.

According to Witley Council rules, a fixed amount of money was deducted from my training allowance for board and lodging. I did not grudge this though, as Hammersmith's Hospital's food was plentiful and there was always a good choice available. The cooks worked very hard day and night to feed the many hungry patients and staff.

Every afternoon, for the first hour after lunch, Miss McLean taught us how to bandage every part of the anatomy. After we worked through the A-Z of bandaging, practising on each other with often hilarious results, bandages were neatly rolled back using an old wooden bandage roller, and this was returned back into a starting position.

The final lectures of the day came after tea break, and a short study period, but by this time, I was so tired it was hard to take much in, despite the flow of air from the constantly opened windows.

At 5.30pm, we were finally dismissed for the day, with corrective tutts of disapproval from Sister Tutor as we filed through the doors.

'Nurse, do straighten your cap…and Nurse, your shoes could do with a good clean. Really!'

Wrapped up in our navy and scarlet woollen capes, we retired to our rooms clutching the day's lecture notes. Lecture notes and numerous diagrams had to be copied and put into my notebook each evening. My notebooks containing hours and hours of written notes would be collected and examined by the Tutors to be returned usually just with a pencil tick. However sometimes the tutors would pencil in the occasional comments such as 'your diagrams are very neat' or worse, 'please see me with this book' in bright red ink.

With so much to learn, the light rarely went off before midnight. I had little difficulty falling into a deep sleep at the end of each day.

A lot of knowledge was crammed into my head over those first three months on PTS, and the hefty schedule certainly pruned out the less determined. Amongst other subjects, our set studied the History, Theory and Practise of Nursing, anatomy, physiology, dietetics, bacteriology, psychology, tray and trolley setting and personal and communal health. My lecture notes even included details about the air ventilation system at the Royal Festival Hall.

My notes from one lecture read, ' *The nurse must look tactfully at the patient's hair in search for lice,*' and the notes then went on to discuss the life cycle of 'pediclosis capitus' a.k.a. the lice. Pubic lice were not mentioned at this particular lecture, but the unsavoury creatures did exist; nasty little things, as we later discovered to our horror.

The male reproductive system was not studied until very late in my training. When the time came, a Mr Grosvenor instructed us. His excellent lecture would still be considered very prudish and incomplete by modern standards.

Coming from a convent school, I was as green as a cabbage as far as sex was concerned. 'O' Level biology had included studying the reproductive works of the rabbit, and so I assumed humans were similar. Before Mr Grosvenor's lecture, however, I had managed to glean a little more knowledge on sex by asking the Librarian in the Hammersmith Public Library for a book hidden from public view amongst the so-called 'dirty' books. Blushing furiously, I had felt it important to inform the stern looking male librarian I was training to be a nurse. After my explanation, his look of disapproval immediately vanished, and the librarian couldn't do enough to help me.

One special lecture given on PTS that had me enraptured, was given to us by Dr. Fletcher, later to become a Professor in his field. Complete with graphic gory illustrations of the diseased blackened lungs from a patient, this great man put most of us nurses off cigarette smoking for life.

For most of the girls on the Set, Dr Fletcher was presenting completely new information. In the 1950s, smoking was actively marketed as a glamorous lifestyle, and little had then been made aware to the public of its harmful side effects. In May 1956, RH Turton, The Government Health Minister, rejected calls for a government campaign against smoking, saying ill effects from smoking had not *actually* been proven yet.

Leading British tobacco firms such as Imperial Tobacco, also issued a statement in the light of The Medical Research Council's report that stated heavy smokers had a twenty times greater risk from dying from lung cancer than non-smokers, but Imperial Tobacco et al claimed,

> *'The evidence of the possible relationship of lung cancer and smoking is conflicting and very incomplete; much more research is necessary before firm conclusions can be drawn.'*

The tobacco firms continued, that certain *'statistical inquiries'* could not be used as conclusive evidence, and pledged £250, 000 towards further research. Their statement brazenly concluded,

> *'Tobacco is a great boon to many millions of people in this country and throughout the world; the benefits, psychological and physiological, it may confer are not yet fully understood and might well be the subject of investigation.'*

In the meantime, Dr Fletcher's graphic evidence was all that *I* needed to make up *my* mind as to the health risks of smoking.

After a few weeks into the course, our PTS were bussed off to Invalid Cookery classes each Thursday afternoon. Crammed into a tiny space at the Addison Gardens Institute, all of us hot and uncomfortable in the August heat, we learnt how to make junkets, egg custards, jellies that would never set because of the heat, and beef teas. I ate what I made, and however wobbly my jellies looked, they actually tasted quite nice.

Over the months, we had a few educational afternoon excursions that were a great diversion from the 'talk and chalk' – trips to a rubbish-sorting depot, a sewage works, and to the Royal Festival Hall to see their modern ventilation units. Glaxo and The Express Dairy gave us superb free teas when we visited them, and I hope their staff received wonderful care from us in lieu.

Fridays always brought the dreaded one-hour practical test. Throughout our training, we were each allotted a bed-making partner. Shirley was my partner, and in the afternoons before suppertime, we practised making up the various beds such as an operation bed, a plaster bed or an admission bed complete with hospital corners. Many a happy hour was spent in the practical room practising making all kinds of beds, while bitching about various staff members, usually Miss Smythe-Jones.

Throughout all the training, it was instilled in me that everything had to be exact, and just 'so' and it was not for me to question 'why?' at any time. For example, every single item had to be carried around on a tray or trolley, never by hand. My small fully indexed Tray & Trolley hardbound notebook, listed seventy-two trays and trolleys, all of which needed to be learned by heart.

For instance, a 'Taking temperatures tray' required glass thermometers in carbolic solution, a wristwatch, white cotton-wool swabs, and water, each demanding its own separate stainless steel kidney dish on the tray. Finally, a pen and ink and an empty dish for dirty swabs were placed on the tray.

There was a lot to learn, and more numbers dropped from our set. Some girls didn't leave because of the harsh discipline. Some left just because they were homesick. I was sad when both the Welsh girls left after just a few weeks in London. Both from the 'Land of song' with beautiful voices, I loved to hear them sing 'All through the night' in their rooms. But they found noisy, smoky London too strange after their lush, gently rolling green valleys.

Very conspicuous in our white attire, bit by bit, those that remained on the Set learnt the ways of the staff, and the ways around the massive buildings of Hammersmith Hospital.

We led a rather 'cloistered' existence. Miss Butcher, the Home Warden looked after the mail from home that kept us up-to-date with life outside Hammersmith's walls, carefully distributing it in pigeonholes behind a foyer opposite the nurse's sitting room.* A night pass was occasionally issued, to permit us to stay out until 11pm; otherwise, 10.30pm was the lock-up time. There were a few rebels who would find a way back into the Nurse's Home long after curfew, by climbing in through windows, after a 'leg-up' from their obliging boyfriends. Personally, I did not see where these nurses got the energy from to go out anyway. In addition, this was a very risky business, as Matron Godden and Principal Tutor Miss Smythe-Jones, were known to lurk around Hammersmith House ready to pounce on any unfortunate late-comers.

On the few occasions I left the hospital premises over those months, I always got a cheery nod and wave from the Head Porter on the Gate, Mr James. He was one of the hospital fixtures and fittings, having been on the gate for many years. He loved his job and his hospital, and he saw all the comings and goings from his post. He was ever vigilant, being the first person to see a patient in, and the last person to see a patient leave, solemnly removing his cap every time an undertaker's van passed out through the gates. He took the trouble to learn all the nurses' names, and his ready smile and kind blue eyes cheered many a weary nurse. He never 'grassed' any nurse up if he saw them sneaking in late at night. Mr James was on our side. It was nice to have at least one ally at the hospital.

Once a month, came Payday. We all trooped up to the Admin. Office, in our time off, and queued up for up to an hour on tired, aching legs for the cash payments. The first month after tax and NI, and board and lodging, I received about £6. Each year, my meagre allowance increased slightly as the student nurse needed even more supplies of textbooks, exam fees, and

---

* Staff nurses had their own, much posher, sitting room, and Sister did even better - but we mere mortals never got a peep behind this 'holy of holies'. It was of course beneath their dignity to eat meals amongst us, so Sisters also had their own dining room.

stockings and shoes that so quickly wore out.

During the last four weeks of PTS, we were each sent up to a ward to do an afternoon in readiness for the first placements after PTS. My assigned ward was B5. 'Sister Fowler's not so bad there,' I was told, but some unfortunate girls from our set were sent to some real dragons. I soon learned, however, it wasn't just the Sister we had to keep on the right side of. Staff Nurses, too, could make our lives a real misery.

Our final PTS exam drew near. Long written papers and practical exams were taken under the beady eyes of Queen Bee, Matron Godden, herself. Our Practical exams included having to lay up a tray or trolley. The day before the exams, every contraption, instrument and piece of tubing was polished, cleaned and laid out on sterile white cloths by us students, while we desperately tried memorising what was what and its uses.

From a grizzly array of shining stainless steel instruments, Matron picked up a Doyen's mouth gag and asked me its function. Standing to attention, with my hands clasped behind my back, I shakily replied, quoting its textbook description.

'Make me up a tray for passing the flatus tube, please, Nurse.' Matron then asked. Luckily, I remembered all the necessary items and laid up the tray in the expected nick of time.

'Trolley for a patient's bath, Nurse.' Matron commanded next. The top shelf had eleven requirements including nail scissors, nailbrush, bath thermometer and two flannels all requiring their own separate receiver or enamel kidney dish. The lower shelf included two bath blankets, two clean sheets, hot water bottle in cover and a 'tray with a drink'. The last shelf needed a small mug, cold-water jug, hot water jug and a soiled linen container. Once again, I got it done in the expected time.

'I would like a bandage to the left eye now please, Nurse'. Eye bandages were not the easiest to apply, and probably through nerves, I applied the difficult roller bandage back to front.

Shirley and I were then given an amputation bed to make up at our bed-making examination, which we did in around two minutes flat.

The whole practical element of the exam took a frantic quarter of an hour per nurse. On the wards, patients' lives depended on the speed to which we carried out our duties, as we were often reminded by Sister Tutor with sharp barks on PTS.

My PTS days were drawing, thank goodness, to a close, and soon I would be let loose on my first ward. A curt letter from Assistant Matron's office invited me to go to the sewing room to be individually measured up for a grey uniform dress for the next stage of my training. Forty of us were invited by Matron up to the Sewing Room. Seven girls had already left, and we were only three months into the three-year course.*

Matron Godden and Principal Tutor Miss Smythe-Jones came out at 10am on the final day of PTS, giving an overly long talk, before finally putting us all out of our misery and disclosing all forty of us had passed the exams. I breathed a huge sigh of relief. I could have kicked myself though, when I was told I would have come first in class, had I not made the mistake of putting the eye bandage on back to front during Matron's exams.

I was pleased that Shirley, Claire and Trudy had made it this far with me. Another girl, Susan, I had become friendly with, had left in tears just days before finals.

I looked around the sea of relieved faces wondering how many of them would still be here this time the following year. Would I? I wondered. Who knew?

---

* Despite Hammersmith's reputation for hard training, this dropout rate was comparable to other hospitals of the era.

Doris Day was top of the charts with 'Whatever Will Be Will Be':-

'Que sera, sera

Whatever will be, will be

The future's not ours to see

Que sera, sera

What will be, will be'

How true! But I was determined to stick the training out come what may, to prove to Miss Smythe-Jones, my family, Ginger and all the other mockers what I was made of.

A big party marked the end of the June 1956 PTS. We celebrated by making lots of cakes and jellies, and I made water lily serviettes to adorn all the tables. All the tutors joined in our celebrations, although some, as expected, never actually let their hair down. Did they ever have fun, I wondered?

PTS had been very tough going, but as they say, 'you ain't seen nothing yet.

CHAPTER IV
Onwards And Upwards...

I went home for the weekend. It was lovely to see my family and Ginger, whom I made a great fuss of, but I expect I smelt a bit hospitally to him as he sniffed curiously around me. Even though I had been away for such a short time, there was a marked contrast between home and my new life just seven miles down the road.

That Saturday night, I went dancing with some girlfriends down the Kensington Town Hall for what was known as the 'Hop'. As I dressed up for the night out, I felt like I was coming out of Purdah. I put on my favourite dress, a pretty floral cotton button-through number that Mum had run up for me on her sewing machine. Underneath this, I wore several layers of petticoats, as was the fashion. A pair of high-heeled white shoes and some little faux pearl earrings and a matching choker necklace I'd been given for my eighteenth birthday completed the look. Puckering up in the hall mirror, I added a touch of eye-blue and lipstick, and made the final adjustments to my hair. A pretty young woman smiled back at me. Yes, and that's indeed what I was! Not just a 'thing' to be shouted at, bullied and ordered about!

A dab of my favourite perfume, Coty's Muguet de Bois, made a welcome change to the stench of hospital disinfectant. I was now looking and smelling human again, and ready to hit the dance floor.

Kensington Town Hall was a different world from the hospital, and it was so nice to be asked to dance by polite young men and be taken through slow foxtrots, waltzes and the more difficult quickstep, to crooners singing Frank Sinatra or Dean Martin numbers. I loved Ballroom dancing, and in the darkened hall with the glistening mirrored ball reflecting light around the room to the stirring rhythm, it was easy to momentarily blot from my mind the past few months.

Many of Hammersmith's youth met their life-long marriage partners waltzing away. I chattered with my girlfriends, as we breathlessly compared our dance partners, wondering if each one might be our very own Mr Right.

'Do you come here often?' came the frequent line.

'Well…actually no!' I could honestly reply.

'That bloke over there fancies you! He's a nice bit of stuff, Cynthia!' Anne giggled.

'And that funny looking one with glasses has been staring at you all evening!' added Carol, throwing in her two-penny worth.

'I don't fancy either of them!' I laughed.

Unlike the last two generations of women, my girlfriends and I could be relatively picky with our men. A time of relative peace, and a rising birth-rate meant a far bigger 'sea' to fish men out of.

National Service was a bit of a pain though. I'd quite often find that a bloke I met was on his last night of freedom, before joining the six thousand other reluctant conscripts that were sent out each fortnight, to do two year's compulsory National Service. It was a real nuisance for me! But at least the men returned alive, and there were still plenty enough men to go around for us girls in the meantime.

I loved looking feminine in a pretty frock and layers of petticoats and high heels, but for every girl who dressed like me at the dancehalls there was another girl in a sweater, jeans, flat ballet pumps and with her hair tied back in a pony tail. When a girl could pick and choose her dance partners, she need not spend so much time getting dressed up.

Most of the men had a 'short back and side's' haircut, and wore rather conservative looking dark coloured suits with crisp white shirts and

42

ties. There were a few men who dressed like Teddy Boys, with the heavily oiled quiff at the front and the obligatory 'DA' and long sideburns, but I steered clear of them, having been warned they were the 'bad boys'.

The Teddy boys dressed to shock, and were a symbol of the working class angst of the youth of the fifties. Their clothes which entailed reams of excess material was a loud rebellious statement against clothes rationing which was still in existence when they'd first appeared on the scene, two years before, in 1954.

An article in 'The Family Doctor' magazine commentated, 'When *any sex is outnumbered at the mating season, it will seek to attract by personal adornment. This is now finding expression at the adolescent level in terms of the Edwardian suit. ...There is no doubt that modern young women like the Edwardian fashion. The evidence is clear in any dance hall.'* *

The Teddy Boy's exuberant dress code certainly made a marked contrast to the male fashion of the time. The 'Teds' attired themselves in patterned silk waistcoats over frilly shirts, over which were worn long, colourful, Edwardian style drape jackets with black velvet lapels, cuffs and pockets. Around their necks hung a tie - usually of the 'Slim Jim' or bootlace variety. Narrow 'drainpipe' trousers, the tighter the better, jived the night away as nimble feet dressed in loud fluorescent coloured socks, worn under pointed winkle-picker shoes completed the look.

The women on their arm usually wore toreador trousers or circular 'poodle' skirts, with low cut tops.

Because of their reputation for violence, youths wearing 'Edwardian dress' were beginning to get banned from entering many places. 'No Edwardian clothes please' signs hung firmly in cinema doorways. After the showing of the film 'Blackboard Jungle' which featured Bill Haley's 'Rock

---

* Dr J. McAlister Brew, writing in the BMA publication, 'Family Doctor' 28/06/1955

Around the Clock' jive music (or 'jungle' music to fundamentalist preachers), the Teddy Boys had got themselves a bad name.

Earlier that September, police had been called to various cinemas showing 'The Blackboard Jungle' in Shepherd's Bush and Kilburn to control the crowds of 'very excited youth'. The Teddy boys and girls 'crime ', it seemed, was that they had started clapping hands and banging their feet to the music and as the tempo grew faster, they'd left their seats to dance in the cinema aisles. Over the other side of the Atlantic, many had condemned Bill Haley's music for the very same reason: it shockingly inspired fans to leave their seats and dance in the aisles.

Clashes had only occurred when the cinema management had tried to get the rocking and rolling Teddy boys and girls to leave the cinema mid-film. The Teds had ripped out the cinema seats and there was a bit of hustle as protesting fans were ushered out. The clashes were relatively minor, but received a lot of bad press.

Still, the Teds behaved when they were allowed to do what they were best at; dancing. The Teds were a colourful sight on the dance floor, dancing wildly to Rock and Roll music or doing the jive, where the girl was hurled in the air or flung at speed through her partner's legs. They certainly stood out from the more sedate 'swingers' like me dancing to Sinatra and the other crooners!

I did not want to be flung about, so politely declined any offer of a dance from one of these male peacocks. There were luckily plenty enough offers from the other men.

Some of the men would know who the Student Nurses were, and would make a beeline for them, and only them, as soon as the first number beckoned us 'boys and girls' to the dance-floor. This caused catty comments and evil eyes from the shop girls. Men seemed to find it very appealing to

44

date a nurse. They probably thought they would get well looked after.

'Men are generally big babies and love to be mothered,' was one of Mum's pearls of wisdom. Her other favourite saying was, 'Kissing don't last, but cooking do.'

Some of the men, I am sure, had a nurse fetish, although I was very young and naïve and knew nothing about those sort of things then. I did enjoy the extra attention and took it at face value. A nurse very rarely needed be without dates in those days. That is, if she had the aptitude and energy for it!

The appeal of dating a nurse would very soon wane for most of these men after constantly being kept hanging around waiting for us to come off shift. This and not being able to see each other often, or at 'normal' hours, meant it was very hard work being a nurse's beau. Those hardy men who persevered in spite of these obstacles, usually found his nurse girlfriend too tired to do anything much on the eventual date anyway.

Although I didn't meet anyone special at 'the Hop' that night, I had a wonderful evening, and returned home from the dancing glowing, on a high, still humming 'La Mer' to myself. I had a blissful Sunday morning lie-in to look forward to.

~ ~ ~ ~ ~ ~ ~ ~ ~ ~

I spent a very lazy Sunday, sleeping in late and then catching up on all the gossip with my younger sisters, Diana, Lucille and Madeleine. Our family had not long finished Sunday supper, comprising of one of Mum's infamous Shepherds Pies, when there was a knock at the front door. A good looking, fair-haired young man, from the nearby Roman Catholic Church, was asking all the local parishioners to join the 'Legion of Mary'. My mother considered it rude to talk to anybody on the doorstep, and so invited him in.

The young man's name was Patrick, and as he sat in our front room, he explained his mission to our religious family. I noticed him looking at me more than once, and I quickly realised that the gorgeous young 'missionary' had taken a fancy to me. There was something about Patrick's blue eyes that I found very intriguing. Unfortunately, I could not stay longer to talk as long as I would have liked, as I had to hurry back to the hospital. I was to be on duty the next morning on my first ward at 7.30am.

'Bye, Mum,' I kissed her cheek quickly, brushing past the seated stranger.

'Bye, Patrick.' The stranger smiled at me. He was even more handsome when he smiled.

~ ~ ~ ~ ~ ~ ~ ~ ~ ~

The feeling of blissful normality left, as soon as the Head Porter, Mr James, waved me back through the Hospital gates. As I unlocked room 207, and plonked myself wearily on the bed, I wondered what the rest of my training had in store for me.

Any naïve optimism that I'd got through the worst block of nurse training on PTS was soon banished, as reality hit me full in the face on the wards. With so much 'dirty work' and cleaning to do, usually two girls fresh from PTS were sent to each ward. I was assigned to Ward B5 with Janet, a small, dark-haired girl from Norfolk.

'On duty, Sister.' Janet and I reported in unison, to the Sister of Ward B5, dead on the stroke of 7.30am the next morning. Janet and I were already a little familiar with B5, after spending four afternoon placements there during our last weeks on PTS.

B5 was a ward of the 'Nightingale' type design, treating men with chest illnesses. The floor was polished like a mirror. Twenty-eight beds with pale green counterpanes pulled into crisp hospital corners, all stood neatly lined up opposite one another, with the exact same space between each one.

Bed lockers were placed with exacting military precision between each bed, ensuring that no patient encroached even an inch onto the other patient's territory. Each bed had its gleaming wheels turned inwards.

Large and lumbering screens had to be wheeled around the wards to give patient's privacy. These, like shopping trolleys, tended to have a life of their own, generally deciding to go in the opposite direction to which they were being pushed. They were also rather noisy.

There were two side wards attached to the main ward. These side wards were used as single rooms for patients that were very ill, or by those patients with the money and the inclination to pay something towards already over-stretched NHS funds for privacy. Little by little, charges were beginning to creep into the NHS. Prescription charges of a shilling had been implemented in 1952 - Bevan's dream was costlier than any government could have possibly foreseen in 1948.

Sister Fowler's office had pride of place, overlooking the ward. A clinic room, kitchen, storeroom, linen cupboard, bathroom, sterilising room and 'the sluice' also made up Ward B5's domain. I was soon to become very familiar with the Sluice, as I was to spend most of my time there. Steam hissed from the bedpan washer, and the air mingled with the smell of stale urine, dirty linen awaiting scrubbing, and drying rubber sheets. Gleaming crystal-clear glass urinals and sparkling stainless steel washing bowls, bedpans and enamel tooth mugs stood ready for service on the shelves.

My mind whirring with all my newly acquired PTS knowledge, from bed-making to delousing, I listened to Sister Fowler's instructions. Put succinctly, my duty was to get on with all the dirty work, never question, rush around as fast as lightening and keep out of everyone's way.

The sputum pots' contents needed collecting from each patient, measured, and then reported in a little spiral bound notebook. As Sister

Fowler showed us the procedure, Janet's face went quite white, and she looked as if she were going to vomit.

'Its not a very nice job, but someone has to do it.' Sister explained. Sister nodded at me. 'It needs to be done first thing each morning. Take it in turns.' PTS Lecture notes on the 'Observations of urine, faeces, sputum and vomit' had really not prepared either of us for this ghastly job that the lowest of the ward pecking order had to perform.

Any relief about what either of us had to look forward to on our days off sputum collecting, was short founded. The alternate task was collecting the dirty dressing's bags, cleaning out the dressing's bins and putting new bags in place. 'Not such a bad job,' we'd thought, but frequently these thin brown paper bags collapsed apart, strewing their smelly contents all over the place. Worse, I was never allowed to wear rubber gloves for any tasks, however dirty.

My year's experience as a SJAB volunteer on Tuesday evenings at Hammersmith Hospital had prepared me for some of the ward's sights and smells, but it in no way prepared me for the rudeness or the sheer amount of dirty work thrust at me. Now I was 'signed up', and no longer a 'civvie', the staff felt they didn't have to be nice to me any more.

My time was filled from morning to night with no let-up. There were the endless Bottle Rounds, where I needed to measure and 'chart' each man's urine bottle, followed by the fetching and emptying of the bedpans known as 'beeps' . With no disposable items, all the equipment need to be washed, sterilised and polished until it gleamed after each use.

Bed-making was at least three times daily, early morning, midday and evening, and the dirty sheets were then hand scrubbed by me in the sluice. Complete bed rest was prescribed to many of the men on B5, and this entailed lots of lifting, without the aid of machinery or a burly porter. Bed baths and turning the patient frequently were administered on Doctors' orders to prevent bedsores from occurring. It was all very heavy work.

In between all this, I served meals and drinks, refilled water jugs and arranged visitor's flowers. I would also be expected to collect the rubbish every three hours from all bedside lockers and tables.

Ward work with its draining routines, took most of my waking moments and energy. The little spare time I got was spent sleeping, eating and peeing, and many a time it didn't feel like there was time even for that. As encouraged, I read up as much as possible on various diseases and illnesses in the few odd moments I managed to snatch between shifts.

It was constant rush, continually observed by Staff Nurse Evan's beady eyes. My evening ward experience as a SJAB volunteer had not prepared me for the hectic routines of ward work either. I was soon to realise this was because evenings were usually *far* quieter than the days.

'Hurry up, Nurse Carstairs, there's no time to talk to the patients.' barked Staff Nurse Evans on my first day. Almost running, I rushed between the patients to ensure fluid balance 'intakes and outtakes' charts were up to date.

'You may go to coffee now, Nurse, and be back for 9.45am *sharp*. And, nurse, take these to the Pathology Lab on your way.' ordered Staff Nurse Evans, thrusting a tray with three Universal Container glass specimen jars, with their rather unsavoury contents, into my hands.

I rushed across the yard to H Block. It was a gorgeous autumn day, but on subsequent days, I would not always appreciate the compulsory dose of fresh air en-route to the restaurant. On night duty, I would sometimes have to wade through the snow to get to the dining area, wet and chilled to the bone. My red and navy nurse's cloak was little protection against rain or snow. There were no underground tunnels joining B to H Block then, so trolleys transporting patients were also exposed to the elements.

'How's it going, Cynthia?' asked Claire in the long coffee queue at the restaurant. She looked as knackered as I felt.

'Staff Nurse Evans on B5 is a real bitch … what's yours like, Claire? I've heard your Staff is even worse than mine!' I griped, sharing my first morning's experiences during a precious five-minute sit-down over coffee.

Then it was back to the mayhem of the ward. Staff Nurse Evans pounced, as soon as I entered through the ward doors, thrusting a list of patient's names into my hand.

'Here are the blanket baths for you to do before Doctor's round at 11.30am. Get Janet to help you.' It was easier and quicker for two of us to work together for this task. With Janet pushing, and I pulling, we puffed and panted as we dragged the noisy and cumbersome privacy screens from bed to bed. The patient's bottom was rubbed with soap, dried and then rubbed with methylated spirit followed by a liberal dusting of talcum powder every four hours, and bed baths needed to be given on Sister's orders once a day.

It was then that Janet and I encountered a man's private parts for the first time ever. Nudity was not then commonplace on TV screens or in the cinemas, we had been brought up to save sexual experimentation for marriage, and the male anatomy model back in PTS had been sexless, rather like an Action Man Doll. We both really had no idea what to expect.

As Janet and I blushed and fumbled around, the situation got even more embarrassing when the poor patient got an erection! Rather shocked, I had no idea at all what was happening. In time, I'd learn to think nothing of such incidents, and would coax shy patients to strip, with the encouraging words,

'Don't worry, Mr Jones, I've seen it all before!'

As we completed bathing the last patient on Staff Nurse Evan's list,

50

whiffs of freshly brewed coffee come from the kitchen. The coffee unfortunately wasn't for us, or our patients, it was brewed especially for the Doctors, due on their daily rounds. All needed to be spick and span on the ward for these occasions, taken so seriously by Sister and her staff. Their ward was their badge of honour, their showpiece, and it must sparkle and shine, and be the very best kept in the hospital.

'Nurse,' yelled Staff Nurse Evans to me, 'Did you polish this table today?'

'Yes, Staff!' I replied rushing to pick up a patient's dropped hankie. Staff Nurse Evans flicked at an imaginary fleck of dust on the table she was complaining about. The central ward table gleamed with bees wax and elbow grease; it had to look at its very best for the doctors to put their 'sacred' clinical notes on.

The Doctors pretended we trainees did not exist, and for the most part, ignored us. On the rare occasions they acknowledged me, the doctors looked at me with so much contempt, I quivered, sure I must have trodden in something smelly and disgusting.

As soon as doctors left, it was time for lunch to be served. All the meals were good wholesome food. Before lunch, patients would be made as comfortable as possible, and propped up in bed. Then the large steel trolley that had been plugged into a heat socket was opened, for the mealtime ritual to begin.

Lunch was a great event as Sister Fowler dished out, assisted by Staff Nurse Evans and a Third Year Student Nurse. Sister knew precisely what each patient needed, their individual dietary requirements and appetites, and would adjust for whom she was dishing up for accordingly.

Meals were seen as an important part of a patient's treatment and recovery, and not just as an aside. Great care was taken to make the meals look attractive, ensuring there was a nice variety of colour on the plate from the different foods. We would *never* dish up an 'all white' meal for example of fish, potatoes, and cauliflower.

'Bed one, for Mr Starkey, Nurse.' and taking the tray from Sister, aware of the critical stares directed towards the back of my head, I carefully brought Mr Starkey his hospital dinner. Not a peck of food was allowed to slop over the hot plate, and I delivered the meals under an aluminium plate cover, as, 'Hot food requires a hot plate, Nurse!' I'd help feed any patient if they needed it, and this would mean time to have a cherished few minutes sit-down while doing so.

After dinner, I collected the food trays and took them back to the kitchen. Domestics and orderlies were employed by the hospital, but they were notoriously slow and not to be relied on. They did not see why they should work quickly, and so did not. Their 'work to rule' would often mean that they sat in the bathrooms frittering away time, while we nurses had to rush around doing our work *and* theirs!

In the 1950s post-war boom years, there was a notorious shortage of manual labour, particularly in London, with nobody wanting to do the 'dirty' work. It was hard to get anyone 'good'. As a consequence, we nurses suffered, having to undertake even more duties. The government had attempted to remedy this problem by extensively advertising in the former colonies, inviting people to come over and live in Britain and take the 'dirty' work on. Nursing, also was widely recruited for in this way. The McCarran-Walter Immigration Act of 1952 had paved the way for West Indians to flock into Britain for work, followed by Indians and Pakistanis toward the end of the decade.

Still, with full employment, people of every colour shied away from the dirty work. I could hardly blame them. With labour so hard to come by, it surprised me that Staff were so rude to us student nurses. In retrospect, it surprised me also that so many of us students took their rudeness.

The patients were wonderful to me, they really appreciated all I did for them, and proudly told me all about their families, pointing out hazy figures in black and white snapshots.

'Quick, *she's* coming after you again.' whispered Mr Jackson, conspiratorially. I nodded and quickly slipped the apple that Mr Jackson had just given me in my pocket, as Staff Nurse Evans suspiciously peered behind the screen and ordered me to take another patient to x-ray. My dress had big pockets, fortunately.

My first day was a split shift. This meant Janet would work the afternoon shift, and I the evening. It also meant that for once I had time for a leisurely lunch at 1.30pm, to report back on duty for 5pm. However, my meal was still rushed; I desperately needed my bed. Setting my red alarm clock for 4.15pm, I was soon sound asleep.

Dreams of clanging bedpans and screaming Staff Nurses rattled through my troubled dreams. I awoke still feeling very tired, and with almost every muscle in my body aching.

I walked the corridors stinking of disinfectant, back to Ward B5. En-route, I passed the new set of PTS girls being led in a silent line by Sister Tutor.

'Poor things,' I thought, sympathetically.

There was no need to exchange words with Janet as I relieved her; her appearance said it all. Her face was pale and tired, her hands red and raw, her dress dirty and crumpled, her stockings holed, and her shoes soaking wet as the bedpan steriliser had leaked on her.

'See you tomorrow!' she whispered hoarsely. 'Good luck!'

Thankfully, the evenings were usually a little less hectic, but an emergency admission could happen at any time. I prayed no one else would need a bottle, beep or soil any sheets that evening. My prayers, unfortunately, went unanswered.

At 8.15pm, I asked Sister to go off duty.

'Is the sluice clean, and are all the charts up to date?' she asked, glancing up from her paperwork. The sluice had to be spotless for the night staff hand-over; if the sluice was in a mess, nobody could go off duty, regardless of the time on the clock, the hunger pangs, or the waiting boyfriend.

'Yes, I've checked,' growled Staff Nurse to save my answering, and with a prim nod, Sister granted me permission to go off duty.

As I departed wearily through the ward doors, the words of the lovely hymn 'The day thou gavest, Lord, has ended' echoed through my mind. I left the ward tired, but happy, and proud to have survived my first full day on the wards. It gave me confidence that I would be able to cope with the following two and three-quarter years of training.

I was ravenously hungry, so my supper soon disappeared, as more tales replaying the day's events were shared with fellow students from my set. I hurried back to my room, to get ready for the next day. I cleaned my shoes and then went to have a long hot soak in the bath.

'It's a lovely day tomorrow' by Franc Sinatra blared out from the wireless in Shirley's bedroom.

'It's a lovely day tomorrow, tomorrow is a lovely day,
Come and feast your tear-dimmed eyes
On tomorrow's clear blue skies,
If today your heart is weary, if every little thing looks grey,
Just forget your troubles and learn to say
Tomorrow is a lovely day.'

'What an appropriate tune,' I thought, before switching off the light at 9.30pm. I was soon fast asleep.

CHAPTER V
The World Holds Its Breath

Days flew into weeks on Ward B5. Patients came and went, and the ward routines soon became second nature to me. Quickly, I was to learn that although the nasty plaster model in the PTS classroom was unattractive and gave me nightmares, at least he did not smell and was never sick over me.

New patients arriving on B5 were placed next to the patients that Sister Fowler felt they would get on best with. From the clinical notes she had read beforehand, Sister knew a lot before the patient had even entered the ward. Staff Nurse Evans would introduce the newcomer to his neighbours and explain the routine as she settled him in. The other patients would soon wise him up on the unwritten rules,

'Don't ever ask Staff Nurse or a 'blue belt' (third year student nurse) for a bottle or beep!'

On leaving the ward, the patient's bed was completely stripped down and changed, and every part of the patient's bed and locker, including earphones for the hospital radio, were thoroughly washed with carbolic solution by a junior. Even the silver framed bedstead and the red rubber mattress did not escape the cleaning solution.

It was lovely to wave the cured patients home, but there was also the flipside, and that was seeing some patients die. It was only a matter of time before I had to face one of my patients dying on me. Having a strong religious faith meant that the concept of death did not frighten me, and I realised what a blessed relief it could bring to years of pain and suffering. Saying that, most men on the ward were a little older. When an elderly person passes on, although sad, it feels more in keeping with nature's cycle.

When someone young dies, it is a completely different kettle of fish to deal with.

Some nurses could never face the ordeal. Nora, a pretty bright girl from my set, found her first death so heartbreaking that she quit nursing right away and returned back to 'Civvy Street' in her hometown of Margate.

As I came onto shift one morning, the empty neatly made up bed, and the sad expression on the night nurse's faces, told me straight away that one of B5's patients had died overnight. What was worse; the deceased turned out to be someone I knew personally. My family's postman, Mr Henry, had been 56 years old. He'd been due for discharge later that day, but had suddenly and unexpectedly, died in the night.

Mr Henry was a lovely character, always with a happy smile and a cheerful whistle whilst on his rounds. He'd known my family for years, and remembered me as an excited little girl in pigtails, expectantly watching out our front room window for his arrival on birthdays and other such special occasions.

My immediate thoughts were for Mr Henry's wife and family. Only twelve hours before, Mr Henry had been showing me a snapshot of his little grandson. His family had been busily preparing the house, looking forward to having 'Dad' home with them again. Death seemed such a cruel taunt to the Henry family's built up hopes - instead of welcoming Dad home, the Henry family had the dreaded early morning knock on the door from two police officers.

I wanted to go somewhere private and have a cry, but there was no time, as the living still insisted on being given their beeps, bottles and bed-baths. I was off duty at 1.30pm, so luckily would get the chance then to go the mortuary and say my own goodbyes to Mr Henry.

The mortuary was at the back of the hospital, discreetly hidden far from public view. I rapped on the door, and a rather surprised mortuary attendant agreed to my request to see Mr Henry. Feeling Mr Henry's cold face, I gave him a soft kiss on the cheek and said my farewells. Mr Henry had been 'laid out' lovingly by the night staff, and looked quite at peace.

'Last Offices' was the final duty for any nurse, and was often carried out tearfully. Two nurses were usually involved with laying out each body. 'Laying out' involved washing and grooming the patient's naked body, ensuring that the patient's private parts were modestly covered over with a cloth at all times. Every detail was important, so even the fingernails were trimmed. Respect for the patient's dignity was always uttermost in the nurse's thoughts.

The patient's mouth, nostrils and rectum were packed with cotton wool (as bowel movements could still occur after death and this cotton wool prevented embarrassing leaks), and the patient's big toes were tied together, as was the jaw, before rigor mortis set in. A nametag was attached to the patient's foot, and covering the patient with a white cotton shroud he was placed on a trolley, ready for the porter to wheel him down to mortuary. A purple cover was then placed over the whole trolley. A nurse would always escort the porter and trolley to the mortuary.

The exception to this ritual was where there were special religious requirements concerning care of the body. Gentiles such as myself were not normally allowed to 'lay out' Jews. There were sometime exceptions to this rule. For example, in years to come when I was a trainee Queen's Nursing sister in Kensington, an elderly Jewish lady died from cancer. I had visited her thrice daily, and so had got to know her and her family very well in that time. It has been said that some patients choose when to die, and I believe this was such an occasion. Mrs Schwartz especially held out, waiting for me to be there with her at the time of her death. I was holding her hand as she gently breathed her last. Her family Rabbi afforded me the honour of doing everything at Mrs Schwartz's final end, including the laying-out. This meant a great deal to me.

I was not the only nurse to care enough to attend patients' funeral services off-duty. Sadly, I was to be only mourner at the funeral of ninety year old Rosie McClaren who died whilst I was on Gynae ward. In Rosie's hay day, she had been a dancing Windmill Folie. A great beauty, she had been courted by Society's finest gentlemen. Yet, at the end of her life, no one seemed to care. I requested the morning off, and rushed off on my bike to the funeral in Acton, buying a bunch of daffodils en-route. I was glad I was there to bid Rosie farewell, and to show her someone still cared at her end.

Other patients would usually know of impending deaths of their bedfellows, as the loved-one's relatives came and held their bedside-vigil behind the screens, supported by tea and sympathy from the nurses. The priest or vicar would rush in to conduct his own ritual. In the meantime, Nurse would attempt to keep the patient as comfortable as possible, and made sure he looked his best. A hush would come over the ward, as domestics were asked to stop work, screens were pulled around the other patients, and only the slight squeal of the trolley wheels, the gentle bubble of the sterilisers and the intermittent intercom calls interrupted the respectful silence hanging over the ward.

~~~~~~~~

I didn't manage to get home much, but when I did, Patrick, the good-looking young missionary, always seemed to be there. I think Mum would tell him when I was expected home, and Patrick would just so *happen* to drop by on these occasions with pamphlets or other excuses to do with his Church work.

As Mum busied herself in the kitchen making more tea one evening,

Patrick started to fiddle with his tie nervously, and then coughed a couple of times. He finally came straight out with it, and asked if I would like to go to see 'Swan Lake' with him at the Royal Festival Hall.

'Yes please!' I grinned foolishly. Mum came back in from the kitchen with a knowing smile on her face. Patrick had found out from Mum how much I loved music and ballet, and bought the two 7/6d tickets well in advance so that I could request the day off.

'You lucky cow!' said my sister Lucille, good-naturedly, when she heard Patrick had asked me out. I had my whole family's seal of approval. My family liked Patrick, and well, so did I - a lot!

Despite requesting the time off well in advance, there was no guarantee that I would *actually* get the day off, but luckily, fate was smiling on Patrick and I when Sister Fowler drew up the work rotas for that week.

As I rushed out to meet Patrick on our first date, I felt butterflies in my stomach. We had arranged to meet up for a bite to eat before the ballet at the 'Quality Inn' next to Victoria Station. Patrick had saved up his work luncheon vouchers up in order to get us both a good meal.

Patrick came direct from his work at a Jewellers Shop in the West End, and looked rather suave in his grey city suit. I wore a blue floral cotton 'shirtwaister' dress, and of course a dab of my favourite Coty 'Muguet de Bois'. Patrick treated me like a queen, listening to me intently with an expression of adoration, and for the whole night, I felt like I was walking on air. And that was some feat considering my tired aching legs!

The ballet was wonderful, and as we left the Royal Festival Hall, Patrick slipped his hand around my waist. I could not have felt happier. It was a mild October night, and as we walked along the embankment getting to know each other, a beautiful pair of swans swam gracefully by. I was even happier when Patrick asked to see again, on my next day off. I really wished my day off was the following day, but unfortunately we had to wait another week.

'See you next week, Cynthia,' Patrick whispered softly.

Not even Staff Nurse Evans glowering at me, or Sister Fowler's shouts could take away the high I felt over the next few days at work.

~ ~ ~ ~ ~ ~ ~ ~ ~ ~

There were usually newspapers left around the wards every day, so I never had to buy any, and through these, I caught snippets of what was going on in the outside world. It was fast becoming a very frightening place.

That October and November, the world held its breath over the Suez crisis, and we all desperately prayed there would not be a World War 3. And as the hours ticked by it began to look more and more likely. Petrified nurses huddled, grouped around the wireless, to try and find out the latest information.

In July, Egypt's president, Colonel Nasser, had announced the nationalisation of the Suez Canal Company following Britain and America's withdrawal of financial assistance towards their Aswan High Dam project. The Soviets agreed to provide an unconditional loan towards the Dam project, and at the height of cold war paranoia, the last thing the West wanted was to allow Russia to get a foothold into the Middle East.

The Suez Canal was a key waterway for world trade and an important source of revenue for Britain and France. Big finance, as well as freedom was at stake. Over the summer and early autumn of 1956, events began to look more and more serious, escalating into a full-scale crisis by the end of October. War was inevitably looming, and the Soviet Union threatened to intervene on Egypt's behalf. It was terrifying.

We were all called back into PTS to watch an emergency film on atomic warfare. Horrifying images of death and destruction, screaming and

61

looting burned into my mind. The filmmakers had used data from the Hiroshima and Nagasaki bombings just eleven years before. The film was very detailed and spared no punches, but as a nurse, I had to be equipped with some knowledge to deal with such a terrible event if it arose. Scared-stiff, I along with the rest of my Set prayed desperately I would never have to.

Most of us students were war babies, so had few clear memories of the Second World War that had ended only eleven years before. The Londoners amongst us had been evacuated* to the country, so been saved the

---

* At the age of three, I and my younger sister, Diana, had been evacuated to a large country home in North Wales, belonging to the Hon. Mrs. Roche. She was a kindly woman, although I am sure she was not desirous of her lovely place being filled to the brim with noisy kids from London. Mrs. Roche had had no option though, but to accept the billet office's demands.

Mrs Roche's house had beautiful rambling grounds, with a large lake that we kids used to go fishing on. We were looked after by nuns from the Convent of the Sacred Heart. They had a strong moulding effect on my character. A Sister Guttridge became my surrogate Mum over the war years. I kept in touch with her, and attended the funeral of this wonderful woman when she died at the age of 90 in 2004. Although kind, the nuns were harsh disciplinarians. Punishment for rather trivial things could be a diet of only dried bread and water for a whole day. We were strictly rationed for toilet paper. I remember the nuns doling out the supplies with the catchphrase, 'One sheet for number ones, two sheets for number twos!'

In 1945, I arrived back to the noise and smoke of bustling Paddington Station, bewildered and clutching my little rag doll tightly to myself. A taxi brought Diana and I back to the family home where I was reunited with my mother. We were strangers, I, the chubby toddler had grown into a young girl. I also was introduced for the first time to the three new brothers and sisters that had arrived in my absence!

terror of nightly bombing raids over the City. However, Sister Fowler and
the older members of the staff, still vividly remembered the screaming air
raid sirens, and the deathly silence waiting for the 'doodlebugs' to fall. Some
staff still at Hammersmith had looked after the bleeding casualties that were
brought in from the raids.

Those who were aged fifty or older still had vivid recollections of
both World Wars. Although she did not like to talk about it, Sister Garry
had served as a Red Cross Nurse in the First World War. It was rumoured
that as well as serving alongside Princess Mary, her hair had turned
prematurely white overnight after receiving news that her fiancé had been
killed in action 'somewhere in Normandy'. Like many women of her
generation, spinsterhood had chosen Sister Garry through fate rather than
calling. She had devoted the passion and energies, which in her girlish
dreams were used in marriage and motherhood, to looking after the sick and
dying instead.

As nurses, we were all still dealing on a daily basis with the after-
affects of the so-called 'Great War' every time we emptied a sputum bowl.
Many of our male patients' chest symptoms had begun after surviving gas
attacks in the trenches. But even those seasoned already by world war
admitted that the horrors of *that* war were nothing compared to the atomic
conflict now threatening us all.

On the 29th October 1956, Israeli troops invaded Egypt, and two
days later, Britain and France followed suit, and bombed Egypt. The Soviet
Union was drumming its fingers and getting inpatient, while nervous
patients on the wards reading their copies of 'The Times' twitched.

As the World watched and waited with baited breath, President
Eisenhower flexed his muscles at the UN and pressurised the UK, France
and Israel into agreeing to a cease-fire on the 23rd November 1956. The

Soviet Union then backed down, and the Suez crisis was resolved. Although we technically lost, a nuclear war had been averted. A lot of people went partying that weekend. I didn't though, as my back was hurting too much.

It was now around six weeks into my ward training and I was getting a lot of back pain. Backache, sore feet and chapped hands were par for the course as a nurse, but this felt far more than the nurse's 'norm'. I was reluctant to visit sick clinic and potentially blot my 'copy book' so early on in my training with Miss Smythe-Jones' harsh warning on PTS, 'You are here to nurse and not be nursed' still ringing loudly in my ears.

The pain grew so bad though, I felt I had no option but to report to sick clinic on my next day off. I approached in some trepidation. Luckily, the Staff Nurse in charge of the Sick Clinic in the Nurse's Home was kind, not assuming her visitors were malingerers. Indeed, I had plenty else better to do in my valued free time. I had arranged to meet Patrick for an outing to the Royal Botanical Gardens at Kew.

After a physical examination and then x-rays on my back, I was ordered to go straight to sickbay for two week's compulsory bed rest. Kew and Patrick would have to wait! The sickbay had just six beds and two side wards. It was very strange to be on the receiving end of nursing care and attention; it gave me a completely different vantage point. The clumsy nurse knocking into my bed sent pain juddering up my spine.

Sister Selby, in charge of sickbay, was nearing retirement. She was kindness itself to all 'her girls'. Matron Godden or her deputy visited all of the nurse patients in sickbay on a daily basis to check up on us.

It was a nuisance to be laid up in bed, when I wanted to be doing so many other things. The novelty of bed rest soon wore off after a couple of days. Luckily, Patrick was a regular visitor at my bedside, and kept me stocked up with fruit and books to read, as well as all the latest news.

'It's pandemonium out there, Cynthia.' Patrick panted breathlessly one evening. 'There's queues and queues of cars waiting at the few petrol stations that are still open, and even some blokes standing in line waiting with jerry cans. The government's just announced there's going to be petrol rationing for at least four months, starting from next month, but all the motorists are going mad now and stocking up.'

Since the beginning of the Suez crisis, petrol had been in short supply as fuel supplies coming in from the Middle East had been blocked, causing fuel shortages throughout the whole of Europe.

'Oh my goodness!' I exclaimed, 'What about the medics and other ambulance drivers?' I still vividly remembered rationing. We all did. It had only ended two years before.

'It's alright,' said Patrick, scanning his newspaper, 'Doctors, midwives, and ambulances will be allowed whatever petrol they need.'

'But what if the petrol all runs out?' I fretted.

'It won't run out, don't be silly, Cynth. We're not at war anymore, and in a little while when it all calms down, President Nasser and his chums will want our money again. We'll soon have more than enough petrol to go around again.'

'Maybe...' I mused, not quite convinced.

'It'll be OK. Don't worry about it; just concentrate on getting better.' Patrick's warm hand clutched my fingers tightly.

'He's *so* dishy!' Nurse Barker whispered from the next bed, after Patrick had left later that evening. She was recovering from appendicitis and obviously approved of my new boyfriend. 'I'll have him if you ever get fed up with him! Just pass him on!' she grinned wickedly.

'Tough luck for you, Barker, I'm afraid I'm not planning anything of the sort!' I smiled back.

After one week's bed rest, Dr. (Daddy) Wimbush reviewed my case. Sister Selby and Staff Nurse Mason assisting him on his rounds looked on sympathetically as the great man made his prognosis. Holding up my x-rays to the screen, so I could see the damage for myself, he came straight to the point.

'You have epyphysitis or inflammation of the bone ends, and Schmorl's nodules. The only 'cure' is to give up nursing, or wear a steel corset. I'm sorry.'

I was too stunned to speak. The prognosis came as a crushing blow to me. Daddy Wimbush's words were as judge, jury and executioner. All I could do was cry. Give up nursing? How could I? To me, there was *nothing* else.

That evening, Patrick still clutching the brown paper bag of Cox's Pippins apples he'd brought in for me, looked on sympathetically, as tears of frustration filled my eyes.

'No, I will not give up nursing. I can't. I *must* try, Patrick.' I said, through gritted teeth.

Patrick gripped my fingers tightly and let me sob myself to sleep.

'Whatever happens, I'll be here for you, Cynth.' he whispered softly.

For some people, that would have been enough. For me it was not. Patrick's gorgeous blue eyes, his soft voice, and his strong manly jaw made my insides feel like jelly; Patrick made my world a more special place, but I could not imagine a world without nursing.

Later that night, sleep did not come easily and I had a long chat with the Staff Nurse on duty. Staff Nurse showed me a steel corset and it looked horrible. The 'Waspie' corset I had worn for vanity reasons a few weeks before had been uncomfortable enough.

My sisters Lucille and Diana had giggled as they tied me into a fashionable 'Waspie' corset before my second date with Patrick. It gave me a wonderful shape, accentuating my curves, but boy, was it uncomfortable. I couldn't wait to get out of it a few hours later. I didn't understand how other girls put themselves through this corset torture every Friday and Saturday night. They'd usually compound their suffering by wearing torturously tight winkle picker shoes as well.

Now I was being shown something far worse than a 'Waspie' corset, and being recommended to wear it for the rest of training, which was another two and a half years.

'It sounds bad, Nurse Carstairs, but the decision can only be yours. I feel really sorry for you and I certainly would not like to be in your shoes right now.' Staff Nurse murmured sympathetically.

One of the books Patrick had brought in for me to read was the life story of Helen Keller, born deaf, dumb and blind. Her guts and sheer determination inspired me. If she could beat the odds then so could I! I was beginning to feel a lot less pain as the physiotherapy, drugs and bed rest had kicked in. Pumped with painkillers and naïve optimism, and a strong dose of youthful obstinacy, I made my resolve, damning the consequences.

'Hey there you with the stars in your eyes...Hey there you on that high flying cloud,' Sammy Davies Junior crooned on the hospital radio. Was he talking to me?!

Give up nursing? I could not! I would not! And there was no way that I was going to wear that steel corset! After two weeks of bed-rest I returned back to work on B5, still starry-eyed, albeit minus a steel corset.

CHAPTER VI
'Oh, Come All Ye Faithful'

Christmas was fast approaching, and many staff members told me how wonderful each Christmas was at Hammersmith Hospital.

As Seasonal preparations gathered momentum, any odd spare moments would find me or another girl busy in the linen cupboard, making paper lanterns or pretty chains from coloured rolls of crepe paper. Some nurses like Trudy had great skills in transforming paper into great works of decorative art. Exquisite flowers and swans ensued from her nimble fingers, and made my simple efforts look rather sorry by comparison.

Strict hospital rules, put in place to prevent dust and infection, meant that Christmas decorations could not go up until Christmas Eve, and must be taken straight back down again on December 27th. For just three days, each ward was transformed into a magical winter fairyland by giggling nurses, but the fact that the decorations were only up for such a short time just made Christmas feel that bit more special and exciting for staff and patients alike.

Each Christmas Eve was a hive of activity as nurses rushed around dressing the ward in time. There was great competition between the different wards for the best decorative theme and scenes. Even off-duty nurses came in, attempting to make *their* ward, the loveliest ward in Hammersmith, not to mention London.

Patients watched on in delight, as coloured lights and sparkling tinsel, lightly scented pinecones and sprigs of holly all sprang up and brightened the normally sterile surroundings. Even the sluice was not forgotten, with a cheerful adornment of tinsel lined up in front of the bottles

68

and beeps.

Plenty of food and even some alcohol helped to relax the strict ward routine just a little. Sister Fowler played Santa, stuffing a stocking for each patient full of little gifts, including the obligatory tangerine. Sister then carefully placed nametags on each stocking, in preparation for one round of hers that all the patients actually looked forward to.

Carol singing started from the Hospital Entrance Hall. As the clock tower struck nine at night, following Hammersmith Hospital's Christmas Eve tradition, Matron Godden and her entourage led off the long procession of carol singers, assembled in strict nursing pecking order.

Clutching our carol sheets and pretty glass lanterns, we students, our nurse's cloaks turned inside out to display their scarlet red linings, followed behind the Staff Nurses. The cape had initially become part of the nurse's uniform during the First World War, when military nurses wore short, shoulder-covering cloaks that bore their rank badges or stripes. After the war, these capes were adopted by civilian nurses to be part of their ordinary uniforms. Although the capes looked nice, they were more for show than practicality, and didn't keep the rain or snow from soaking through to our short-sleeved dresses underneath.

We carol singers trooped around the hospital, ensuring every ward was visited on our tour. Nobody, from the very young to the very old, was allowed to miss the visual treat. Matron led us from ward to ward, beckoning us to dim the lights of our lanterns at each ward entrance before we sang our piece.

Matron Godden chose a carol that she felt would suit each ward. A men's ward would hear a hearty 'Good King Wenceslas', and a Maternity ward would hear 'Silent Night' sung in hushed tones.

As I walked and sang, I was acutely aware that I was treading the same path that many Hammersmith nurses before me had walked on this Holy Night, and that many nurses after me would tread. All over the country, I knew, similar scenes were taking place on other wards in other Hospitals too.

There were many wards to visit, and by now, my legs and feet were swollen and aching. I'd already been on my feet all day after working a full shift, but the delight on all the patient's faces more than compensated for this. Arriving at ward B5 was very special for me.

'There's my nurse!' boasted the fragile Mr Bell to a fellow patient, spotting me in the scarlet coated ensemble. Mr Bell knew that this was the last Christmas he'd ever see. Most days, he sat propped up in bed by pillows, blankly staring into space, just waiting to die.

Despite the festive atmosphere, life and death did not stand still within Hammersmith's walls. Patients were still being admitted, and patients were still entering or leaving the world.

Over in the maternity section, babies were being born, and the first Christmas baby, usually nicknamed 'Holly' or 'Noel' by the nurses, was the centre of attention. On another ward, a dying patient was being 'specialled' by a night nurse behind a screen, the Duty Sister dreading having to break the news to his relatives at such an otherwise happy time.

Over in Casualty, road victims were being stretchered in. Some of them had fallen foul to a drunken driver's failing concentration, but many had fallen foul of a far worse enemy. Bad Smog was reducing visibility to virtually zero in some parts. The smog was an annual event, expected by Londoners, but this year the filthy freezing fog caused chaos all over the nation, and lasted for days. The smog had been so bad that December that the Post Office had issued a statement warning the public to post their Christmas cards in plenty of time, or else they could not be guaranteed to reach their destination in time.

When every ward had been visited and I'd sung myself almost hoarse, I went back to 'Hammersmith House' where Mr Banbury, the catering officer, had laid out a gorgeous buffet supper for us all in the nurses' sitting room. I was so tired by this time, it was hard to do it any real justice, but out of courtesy to Mr Banbury, I did my best!

I was to be on duty the next day from 7.30am through to 8.15pm so bed beckoned.

'Goodnight, girls, Happy Christmas!' I yawned, heading back to Room 207.

'Happy Christmas, Carstairs!' There was no need for the others to wish me to 'sleep well'. I was already almost asleep on my feet. Sleep came within minutes of my head touching the pillow.

~ ~ ~ ~ ~ ~ ~ ~ ~ ~ ~

I awoke on Christmas morning, wishing first I was at home with my family, second that I was with Patrick, or third, that I was on duty on children's ward. Every nurse wanted to be on Children's Ward on Christmas morning. To see the excited little faces light up, despite their pain and suffering, was something very special indeed.

Night nurses had crept around in the hush of night placing filled stockings of a little toy, crayon and book at the end of each child's bed. Later, Father Christmas made an appearance, jovially played by the Paediatrician, Dr White. Santa handed out further toys, to squeals of excitement, from his special sack of gaily wrapped gifts generously provided by hospital staff.

I reported on duty to Ward B5, and as I walked through the ward doors, Staff Nurse Evans actually greeted me with a smile. The white-faced dragon could look almost pretty when she smiled. All the Staff went out of their way to be a bit more human to the students on this special day; there

71

was plenty of time to return back to their usual bitchy selves after Christmas was over, after all! The little tipple Sister Fowler had drunk had probably helped loosen her up somewhat too. As a special exception to the Hospital rule, staff were all allowed a little drop of alcohol.

All the ward staff enjoyed a sit-down cup of real brewed coffee, a real treat, as Sister Fowler handed each nurse a present. She gave me a Nursing Mirror Diary. We in turn had been *obliged* to donate to Sister's present, and the princely sum of two shillings had been extracted from each of us for Matron's present. Matron Godden must have done very well indeed out of us all.

Beeps, bottles and treatments continued, but the ward was less full (most patients were sent home for the holiday season if they were up to it). Each bedpan was brought to the patient complete with a sprig of holly; by a nurse wearing a jolly paper party hat that had popped out from the box of Woolworth's Christmas crackers that one patient had got his wife to bring in for us.

For two days even Staff Nurse Evans forgot to chase me. The 'magic bottle' thankfully continued to work its merry magic on her.

The kitchen staff had worked extremely hard since the crack of dawn, and sent up a beautifully cooked turkey with all the trimmings, roast vegetables, plum pudding, custard and scrumptious mince pies to each ward. Surgeons, complete in operating garb, came and carved each turkey for us. The surly men, more used to throwing things at nurses than passing things to them, were all smiles. The bottle, no doubt, had worked its wonders on them too! Professor Jones came and wished us all a very merry Christmas, not forgetting to give Sister Fowler a kiss under the mistletoe.

After serving Christmas dinner to our patients, there was plenty enough for us nurses to have a sit down meal. We all had a wonderful dinner on the patients' leftovers. I think, on reflection, Mr Banbury must have known how many patients to cater for and deliberately added extra for the nurses.

Sister had prepared the dinner table for us nurses beautifully, and it looked a real treat. Our 'official' Christmas Dinner was still a few days later, where by tradition, the Sisters bit their tongues and waited on us. This was the event where Mr Banbury the Catering Officer always carried in the huge Christmas pudding flamed alight with brandy, in another special Hammersmith tradition.

Christmas Day Dinner was followed by a monster wash up. As Janet washed, and I dried, we speculated as to what the year 1957 would hold for both of us.

'Well, I'm not quitting training, that's for sure,' I said, clutching the hospital issue tea-towel more tightly.

'Me neither!' determined Janet, 'If we can cope with Evans we can cope with them all, right, Cynth?'

'Right!' I nodded firmly.

I had high expectations for 1957.The gloom of the Suez crisis was at last behind us, and our young Queen was ruling a new Elizabethan era that seemed full of hope and promise. And then there was Patrick. I sighed deeply, as I remembered his gorgeous blue eyes. Yes, and then there was Patrick.

Christmas Day 1956 was a magical day. When I returned to the Nurses' Home, I found a note pinned up for me on the board to say that Patrick had called to wish me a Happy Christmas.

'And a Happy Christmas to you too, Patrick.' I murmured, as I flopped onto my bed and promptly fell asleep.

CHAPTER VII
A Long Hard Night

Three months had passed since starting my ward duties, and now the rotas were due to be changed. We always had a clear three days notice of changeover. On Wednesday at Twelve Noon, one of the assistant matrons posted up the change list. There, hung my fate for the next three months.

As I eagerly scanned the list for my name, I noticed I had been assigned to ward D2, a female surgical ward. This was a lighter ward than B5, but Sister Shaw was said to be awful there.

As we students compared notes as to who had been given the worst wards, and the worst Sisters, so tongues had been wagging about each of us in the Sisters' dining room. Even before any of us had crossed her sacred threshold, Sister had already formed an opinion on her new minion based on the dining room gossip. Cruel words were spoken about us, and written on reports that we were never allowed to see. Sisters dug the knife in for all manners of reasons, and could ruin many a nurse's life, just because Sister did not like a girl's face.

Not one of my set envied my posting, even Shirley who was replacing me as Staff Nurse Evan's new cannon fodder on B5. Margaret from our PTS set had quit nursing just before Christmas. D2 had been her first ward, and she'd had enough of Sister Shaw's tongue, and the disgusting work thrown at her. She vividly described the mastectomies and colostomies, and how she'd been physically sick in the sluice after emptying her first ileostomy bag.

'Tough luck, Cynthia!' said Trudy pulling a long face, as she waltzed off to C2, the Gynaelogical ward. It was all too easy for her to say!

At least my new grey uniform dress had now arrived, that I'd been measured up for at the end of PTS, and had been eagerly waiting for ever since. Finally, I could ditch the white dress and the stigma of 'PTS girl' once and for all. The change of colour dress was an indication that albeit slowly, I was climbing the nursing hierarchy ladder. Two girls fresh from PTS would now be beneath me in the hospital pecking order, but I would still be known and treated as little more than a raw junior.

Assistant Matron had written to each of us a week before, instructing us to go and collect our new uniforms from the sewing room. The sewing room was approached by clambering up an old iron staircase that clung like a fire escape to the old grey hospital walls. There, the friendly chatter of the Singer treadle sewing machines frantically altered the blue, white and grey nurse uniforms, or repaired the bed sheets, doctor's white coats, and patient's operating gowns. Like the laundry staff who worked in steaming hot conditions, this dedicated team of sewing ladies happily gave a lifetime of service to their hospital.

I was handed three dresses of a dreary grey colour, fourteen white cotton aprons and four white cotton hats. Luckily, I was spared the discomfort of having to wear stiff starched collars. The uniforms were dull and less than glamorous, but it was great to be finally out of the conspicuous white attire of a PTS trainee.

As soon as Claire, Shirley, Trudy and I got our next block of free time, we ventured out to a photographer's studio, where we proudly posed in our new uniforms for some 'polyfotos'. For 7/6d each, we got forty different black and white head and shoulder portraits. I gave a couple to Patrick, and he gave me a picture of him sun-kissed and grinning at the end of Southend pier. I treasured the snap, and put it in my drawer alongside my pictures of Ginger, my girl guides troop and home. I determined to keep my head down and nose clean, and to get through my time on D2 without drawing any more attention to myself. Most of my time on D2 seemed to be spent in the Sluice, so this was relatively easy. I just had to cross my fingers that my back would not let me down in the meantime.

Sister Shaw was as difficult and hostile as I'd been led to believe, but there were definite advantages gained from my move from B5. Far less stress was put on my back, as the women were a lot less heavy to lift than the men, and did not need complete bed-rest. It was also rather exciting to see patients coming and going from real theatre.

On D2 sweet smelling perfume and talc exchanged the smell of the men's 'Imperial Leather' shaving foam and 'Lifebuoy' soap. The patients, as always, were wonderful. Some of these ladies had bravely endured terrible operations, but all were ready to keep an eye-out for us.

'Quick, Nurse Carstairs, Sister Shaw's coming!' they'd warn me, saving my bacon on many an occasion. They really did keep me going when the days seemed so hard, and it seemed I could not do a thing right for Sister. They would often take the blame for an untidy locker or bed-table, and their smiles of encouragement and heartfelt appreciation got me through many a low moment.

'You're doing a grand job, nurse!' and their little gift of a barley sugar, along with their encouraging words, were usually enough to lift my flagging spirits.

One of my patient's on D2 was a Miss Jones. She was furious that her appendectomy had brought her into hospital as an emergency case, as she was one of the few lucky rock and roll fans who had managed to get hold of tickets for the upcoming Bill Haley concert tour. Now, she would not be able to use them.

'It's so unfair!' Miss Jones cried into her crumpled issue of 'New

Musical Express', reading their report on Bill Haley' rapturous welcome to Britain in February 1957.

'New Musical Express', February 1957

'It seemed that half the population turned out to welcome Bill Haley to Britain. As soon as he and his Comets had disembarked from the liner Queen Mary, a chartered train - 'The Bill Haley Rock'n'Roll Special' - whisked them from Southampton to London. All along the route, people waved from windows, stood in gardens and on railway embankments, and hung precariously over bridges. On arrival at Waterloo, the whole forecourt was crammed with over 4000 Haley worshippers, making a noise which rapidly reduced Glasgow's famous Hampden Roar to a whisper. Nobody could do much with that crowd, least of all the police. Once in the middle, Haley's chauffeur driven car was powerless - he was hemmed in for a full 20 minutes while fans clamoured and cheered. But that was nothing compared with the band's opening concert at the Dominion Cinema. You've seen them in their films and heard them on your record players - but how can one possibly describe or explain it, that deafening, devastating EXTRA roar of enthusiasm which greeted and sustained Haley and his Comets that night?'

Bill Haley was becoming a phenomenon - 'Rock around the Clock', the so-called 'anthem of disaffected youth' had sold over one million copies in the United Kingdom, making Haley the first artist ever to win a British gold disc. Youth were deserting swing music by the thousands for the new rock and roll music. I was not one of them, however, and couldn't quite see what the fuss was all about. I had to admit that 'Rock around the Clock' was a catchy little number though, and I found myself humming it from time to time despite myself. Given the choice though, I'd rather dance to Joe Loss's orchestra any day.

'You'll soon be up and about dancing again!' I tried to cheer up my heartbroken patient.

Miss Jones gave me a funny look. I just didn't 'get' it, obviously.

'Oh, you just don't understand!' and Miss Jones started sobbing again into her already tear-soaked copy of 'New Musical Express'.

She was right. I didn't.

~ ~ ~ ~ ~ ~ ~ ~ ~ ~

Approximately one third of my training would be spent working night shift. Each assigned period of nights lasted a full three months, without a break. Each 'night' consisted of a twelve-hour shift. The schedule was five nights on, three nights off, followed by four nights on and then two nights off.

Nights! The very word sent cold shivers down my spine. There was not even the lure of overtime pay to take some of the sting away from it for me. I was warned by enlightened students in the set before me that I would probably get an upset stomach and diarrhoea when starting nights because of the topsy turvy routine. My body certainly found it very hard to adapt to the routine of five nights on, and three nights off, I seemed to be continually out of synch. A few more enlightened hospitals were doing a nine nights on, five nights off system, which in my opinion was much more preferable.

Still, I was lucky in that my first block of nights did not start until April. With the lighter Spring mornings and evenings, I was not having to go on duty in the dark and come off duty in the dark, which I later hated having to do. In the winter, I felt like I imagined a Norwegian living in the Artic Circle felt during one of their winters, seeing only one hour's daylight a day if I was lucky.

The dreaded change list was pinned up once again for all to see. There was no escaping! I just hoped that I'd have a decent Staff or third year student for my first ever block of nights. That would at least make it a little more bearable.

I saw that I was assigned to H6, the male urological ward. I would be expected to interchange with other wards from time to time, but this was my main posting for the allotted time. I breathed a sigh of relief as Staff was alright there; it could have been far worse.

Each Hammersmith ward had its own distinct aroma. H6 was notorious for its stench of urine.H6 was full of mostly elderly men with prostrate problems. This meant a lot of work changing beds and dressings, and turning the patients regularly to prevent bedsores.

My Staff Nurse, Staff Nurse Schroeder, was a middle-aged, exceptionally kind German SRN, with very high standards. She typified German stereotypes, in that she worked like a machine and rarely took any breaks at all.

Clutching my night nurse's bag, containing Tooheys 'Surgical Nursing', some Hardanger embroidery and a clean apron, I was on duty on H6 at 8pm sharp.

Ward Sister was occupied giving her report, escorting Staff Nurse Schroeder on a round, as day nurses busily rushed around them finishing their chores. I was instructed to find my list of duties and to 'get on with it'.

I found my relief slip in the night nurse's drawer. It was a long list of tasks, with a broken down schedule of the times they were expected to be performed at. My first job every evening was to make a goodnight drink of 'Horlicks' or 'Ovaltine' for my patients at 8.30pm, served in a cup and saucer.

After drinks, it was time to hand out the nightly medication. Staff Nurse Schroeder could get her own drugs from the ward cupboard, but needed me to check them with her. She and I then went from bed to bed, dispensing the sleeping pills, antibiotics, painkillers and so on. Dressings were reapplied, pillows were plumped, and the gentlemen were made as comfortable as possible for the long night ahead.

Every patient was always individually wished a goodnight from us. At 10pm sharp, Staff Nurse Schroeder turned off the ward lights,

'Goodnight, boys!' she said in her still noticeably thick German accent.

'Goodnight, nurses!' the patients called back.

That's when the long night would really seem to really start for me.

A green cotton trolley cover was placed over the white Bakelite lamp hanging on the Night Nurse's station, to dim the light even more so as not to disturb the patients. This was my desk, situated around a quarter of the way up the ward, opposite the draughty ward door. From my perch, I had a prime view of every patient. This desk soon had little offerings on it from the patients of fruit, chocolate or pieces of cake.

'Nurse Carstairs, you should not accept anything from the ward, because of the possibility of infection. Really!" Sister tutted in disapproval. These gifts never did me any harm though. Infection was almost unheard of on the wards, as everything was kept so spotlessly clean. But I soon learned to quickly tuck any gift into a drawer away from Sister's eye-line.

On the rare occasions that my Senior, Staff Nurse Schroeder, took a break, she handed me the keys to the Dangerous Drugs cupboard, with strict instructions as to certain patient's care. If Sister wasn't around either, I was left alone in charge of twenty-eight sick men in the darkened ward. It felt very eerie, as cries from the patients mingled with the hissing steam steriliser. Draughts from the open windows would momentarily flick the curtains up an inch or two, so that the moonlight reflected on the glistening floor still smelling of polish.

I found out later, that some of the men on the wards did not have to come at all far to be admitted to Hammersmith Hospital. They came all the way from next door, HMP Wormwood Scrubbs! Had I known on my first night of night duty, that two of my patients were prisoners doing time over the road for 'GBH,' I would have been far more frightened than I actually was. I expect Sister knew our next-door neighbours' history, but had not thought it important to inform me.

Part of H6's treatment regime involved getting bottles and bottles of fluid down each patient, but there were the inevitable consequences of this treatment, as nature played its course. The ward was not nicknamed 'Water Lilies Ward' lightly! Checks on the patients were made by torchlight. The patients rarely asked for a bottle unless they were really desperate and sometimes just sat in their mess until I discovered them. The men would often be terribly embarrassed as they were cleaned up and helped into fresh dry sheets.

'I'm so sorry for bothering you, Nurse.'

'Don't be silly, Mr Adams, that's what I'm here for! Please call me if you need anything. Don't wait so long next time you need a bottle!'

Occasionally the patient would chance their luck and ask me for a cup of tea to help them get back off to sleep.

'You know Sister will have my guts for garters if I make you a cup of char, Mr Adams! Pretend its Horlicks, and I will make you one. Promise?! One sugar or two?' I winked at Mr Adams conspiratorially and returned with a cup of hot tea on a small metal tray. He sipped his tea gratefully, and soon my partner in crime was sound asleep. Tea, the pulling through of a cool clean piece of drawer sheet and the turning over of a pillow really worked wonders.

Although night shifts were always quieter than day shifts, there were still wet beds to strip and change, temperatures to take, blood pressures to monitor and so on. With only two nurses per ward, it was also far harder work as a consequence. My torch flashed on various dials and measuring devices, as I monitored the snoring patient's progress.

Twelve of the men had indwelling catheters collecting their urine. It drained into thick glass Winchester bottles that stood on the floor. These bottles were very heavy to lift, containing twenty-four hours worth of smelly urine that would need testing and charting. The Winchester bottles needed to be thoroughly scrubbed and cold-water sterilised afterwards in the sluice. It was not a pleasant task, but as Sister Fowler had said on my first ward, 'someone has to do it.'

At midnight, huddled under my cape, I made my way along the cold draughty corridors to the staff restaurant for my break. I passed by the night orderly, Don, as he made his own slow, meticulous, journey down the corridors with his bucket and mop. He gave me a big toothy grin; the same smile that he especially saved for all the Hammersmith Nurses.

There was a recreation room I could go to on breaks if I chose. With only three armchairs in the room for fifty of us, it was very much 'first come, first served' as to which lucky nurses had the most comfortable seats at break-time. I preferred to stay in the restaurant chatting with Claire, Trudy and Shirley. It saved my feet more than anything else.

Entering the restaurant, the bright lights dazzled me at first, and it took my eyes a while to adjust from the rest of the dimly-lit, eerily quiet hospital. Enticing smells from the Servery invited me to enjoy a hot dinner. I could not totally unwind and relax even at dinner, as in between gobbled mouthfuls of steak and kidney pie, I had to try to commit my patients' names and their various diagnoses to memory. A slip with this information was in my pocket, that I was expected to learn by heart. It was very hard to commit all the information to memory, however, when the workload was already so hectic.

Peggy from my PTS set, came and plonked herself down beside me with her tray. Peggy was from Leeds and had naturally wavy rich chestnut-brown hair, which I was very envious of. I would have so loved her curls! Instead, nature had given me straight mousy brown hair, and I did not have the time, money or inclination to waste on perming solution.

I liked Peggy; she was a typical no-nonsense Northerner, who got straight to the point. Peggy was fuming, as her Senior had only give her half an hour for break, and this seemed to be the proverbial straw that broke the camel's back for her.

'That's it. I have had *enough*! Why should we nurses do a twelve-hour or more nightshift when Policemen and Firemen only do eight hours for a lot more money? It is ridiculous! What is the Royal College of Nursing supposed to be doing for us, for goodness sakes? I am out of here!' True to her word, Peggy told her Senior where to stick it and left the hospital the next morning. Another PTS girl had bitten the dust! I wondered how many more girls would go before the year was out.

I returned to H6 from my dinner break, and had hardly finished buttoning up my apron, when Staff told me, in no uncertain terms, that there were several wet beds waiting for me, and to 'get on with it'.

I hurried to Staff Nurse Schroeder's command. I had just finished my task, when I heard a patient's frantic call coming from behind me,

'Quick, Nurse, it's Frank, he's falling out of bed!' I managed to run and catch Frank just in time. Frank had a regular habit of falling out of bed for some strange reason, however much I and the other nurses tried to keep him tucked in.

I was able to take a welcome sit-down in the small hours, rolling cotton wool balls and cutting gauze dressings for the stainless steel dressing's drum. From the ward desk, I could see every patient, and I intermittently looked up from my rolling or cutting to check on my slumbering patients.

As I rolled, I tried to recite the patient's names and their diagnosis under my breath, continually trying to run the list through my mind like a mantra so that I would not forget it.

Night Superintendent Thora, on her 2am round, escorted me around my patients one by one, assessing my memory task with arched over-plucked eyebrows.

'Bed One, Mr Adams, day two, Prostatectomy. Bed Two, Mr Smith, day seven, neoplasm of the bladder. Bed Three, Mr Cook, day one, kidney stones...'

I was interrupted by a furious,

'No, Mr Cook is *not*, Nurse! You *must* learn all the names and diagnosis correctly.' There was no way of getting one past Thora. She was as shrewd as a snake and had an excellent memory for detail. She was too clever by half.

Over the coming weeks, I learnt to sprinkle a few Cornflakes on the floor by the door, so Thora's footsteps could be heard, giving me some advance warning of her approach. She had a habit of creeping up very quietly. It was one thing to be quiet, but Thora was *so* quiet that she used to frighten young nurses out of their wits. To suddenly feel a cold hand on my shoulder in the wee small hours, when my imagination was already running overtime, was not pleasant.

Occasionally the other early warning system, the ward telephone, rang, with some kind night nurse on H1 & H2 ward warning me of Thora's immanent arrival.

'Quick! Thora is on the prowl early tonight, so watch it! She's in a filthy mood.' It would be time enough for me to bolt down the rest of my Cornflakes and straighten up my skew-whiff apron.

My tea break was allocated between 3.30am and 4am. I soon learned to use this time for sleep rather than tea. It seemed that I was constantly tired, as not only was work long and hard, but it was so difficult to adapt to the irregular routine brought about by night shift. My body continually seemed to be struggling to play 'catch-up'.

With a senior nurse's permission, I headed to the bathroom with a pillow and blanket from the linen cupboard. There I relieved the previous occupant, and made up my own temporary bed in the empty bathtub, always at risk of being caught out by some less obliging member of staff. Staff woke me up just before the end of my break, and straightening my dress and hat I'd sleepily return back to duty. Failing the bath, the floor of the linen cupboard would serve many an exhausted night nurse.

It was not unknown for nurses to snatch that valuable twenty-five minutes kip on a ward bed. This was even more risky as Night Sister would want the name and diagnosis of the new patient! But many of us regularly took the risk, and thanks to Staff or Senior's vigilance, and the trusty Cornflakes on the floor, the new admission would sleep well, followed by even the Senior Nurse.

Thora was furious with those poor souls she caught in the act, but she was well aware of the practice going on every night under her charge. After all, she too had been a night nurse many years before.

Staff Nurse Schroeder, the German human automaton, never seemed to stop work for any breaks, let alone sleep. Because of her nationality, she encountered silent resentment from many of the men as memories of World

War II were still so raw. Sometimes Staff Nurse Schroeder encountered outright hostility.

'A German?! I'm not being treated by a bleeding Jerry!' spat one Alf Garnett look-alike. An old soldier, it was easy to understand his feelings, but Matron Godden soon put him right.

I think as well as being driven by her inherited national work ethic, Staff Nurse Schroeder felt she had to prove herself by working that little bit harder than anyone else. She had a far harder time of it than any of the black girls, and they had a rough time of it at Hammersmith. Gracie, from Nigeria, was bullied so much because of her colour, by staff and patients alike, she left Hammersmith and England. I had liked Gracie a lot, and was sorry to see her go.

Junior nurses like myself were never allowed to speak to a Senior unless spoken to, so I knew nothing about Staff Nurse Schroeder, what made her tick, or why she had chosen to work in England.

At 4.30am, patients who had been deep in sleep were woken up to have a wash and shave. As cruel as it sounded, we needed to start on the patients early, in order for all our duties to be completed for the day changeover shift at 8am. I crept around from bed to bed with stainless steel wash bowls, and tooth mugs of Glycethylolene mouth wash, and left these on the bed tables of those able to wash themselves.

'You are so cold nurse!' The patients mumbled sympathetically as they felt my icy-cold touch. Whatever the temperature, I was never allowed to wear a cardigan or cape on the wards. My short-sleeved dress had to brave the elements, in front of the constantly opened windows.

Ward domestics did not work at night, so I needed to lay some breakfast stuff out and make early morning tea for the ward. I spread half butter and half margarine onto the brown bread, and the bread was then covered with a damp clean tea towel to keep it from drying out. Proper cooked breakfasts and hot tasty porridge would be sent up to the ward by the Catering staff later on that morning.

My last job, after updating the fluid charts and dealing with even more bottle and 'back' rounds, was to scrub clean all the dirty linen as the sterilisers hissed, and leave the sluice clean and tidy…or else!

After the customary examination of my labours, I was finally given permission to go off duty.

'Goodbye boys!' Staff Nurse Schroeder and I called, as we passed out the doors heading straight for bed.

'Goodbye, Nurses, and thank you!' called back our grateful patients. Then an aching back, supported by aching legs in wrinkled grey nurse's stockings dragged themselves off the ward to a hot bath and bed.

Chapter VIII
Getting A Set Of Wheels

After six months of 'living in' at Hammersmith House, with Matron's permission, I chose to move back home. This had several advantages. The £8 a month board and lodging I had been paying the hospital would help Mum out, I would be amongst my family in more homely cosy surroundings, and more importantly, I should be able to get some much-needed kip during the day. The Nurse's home was in no way conducive to sleeping during the day, with all the banging doors, chatter and blaring radios.

Now it just remained how to get my green trunk home. Petrol was practically unobtainable in central London, even if one had the necessary rationing coupons, and was a resourceful fellow like my cabbie neighbour, Bob Townsend. When Bob did manage to get hold of petrol, he complained bitterly about how he was charged an extortionate six shillings a gallon.

Bob admitted he wasn't the only one hard done by though. Assembly staff at all the major car plants were reduced to working a four-day week, and some poor men had been temporarily put on the dole. Bob's mate, who ran a driving school, Mr Hargreaves, was luckier than many who earned their living by driving. Mr Hargreaves, along with around 700 driving instructors nationwide, was being paid by the government to administer the petrol ration coupons.

I could not afford a taxi fare at the current going rate, and it would not be fair for Bob to feel obliged to subsidise me, like he'd done when he'd first taken me to Hammersmith House, just six months before.

'Don't worry, we'll manage.' said my ever-resourceful Patrick. And together with his strong muscular arms, and the Number 72 bus, that was running even less frequently than normal, we somehow managed to haul my green trunk all the way home.

It was good to be home. Luckily, the rest of my siblings were all out at school during the day, so I had the house pretty much to myself. Ginger came in and curled up into a ball at the end of my bed, and his gentle snores never disturbed me. Our neighbourhood was very quiet and there was little traffic noise, which was remarkable considering we were only five miles from the centre of London. The main neighbour noise was the soft patter of tennis balls on the courts adjoining our back garden, and the occasional cheer or moan as a point was won or lost. Bin day twice weekly with its clanging and banging was hard going, but this could not be avoided.

The disadvantage to moving back home was the distance to and from the hospital. The Number 72 bus was becoming more unreliable and infrequent than ever, and there were long walks for me at each end from the bus-stops. This ate away at my precious free time. Another form of transport was essential.

I scoured the second-hand advert boards, and managed to find myself a sturdy black Raleigh bicycle for £2, 10 shillings. I was very pleased with my new purchase; it proved a fantastic investment, saving me time and bus fares. Cycling also helped keep me fit; not that I needed it though, with all the walking up and down hospital corridors each day.

It was a good time for me to begin cycling in the capital, as the London traffic was down by at least two-thirds. Some of the main streets, normally so noisy and bustling, now felt quite eerie as they were virtually deserted, save for the odd rumble of the trolley bus on the tram lines, or the rush of pedestrian's feet. I pedalled past the boarded-up petrol stations, and the cars lying abandoned at the roadsides, wondering when this silence would all end, and London would return to normal.

My bike proved very reliable, and Patrick was kind enough to fix any punctures, although Mum claimed that Patrick made more punctures than he actually fixed, so as to have an excuse to come and see me. If he did, I could hardly blame him.

Although we had been seeing each other for several months, it had been on rare and sporadic occasions. It was no wonder that at times Patrick felt like a spare part. I didn't want to lose him, but I didn't know how to make it better; I couldn't. Patrick had to take me as I was with all my nurse's baggage, and thankfully his gorgeous blue eyes holding me in a steady gaze, told me he was going nowhere. We had to make every minute count. And as we counted it together, it was precious. Yes, another advantage to being back at home, was I could see my very own 'Mr Wonderful', Patrick, a little more frequently than when I was living at Hammersmith House. Mum's living room was certainly a lot more comfortable than the hospital nookie room!

With the pay left over that month, together with all the rest of my savings, I somehow managed to scrape together £12 and bought myself a navy nurse's gabardine raincoat I saw advertised in the Nursing Times. I was expected to keep my uniform dress covered up at all times if I was outside, so germs from the outside world did not touch my uniform, and thus be brought into the hospital. Before this coat, I'd been changing in and out of civvies. Now I had another time-saver; I only had to get dressed once a day instead of three times. The downside was that I had to keep my coat on even on the hottest of days. I'd arrive at the hospital perspiring, uncomfortable and thirsty, after cycling the seven miles in the beating sun.

On my next night off, after the precious coat had arrived by mail order, Patrick looked very pleased with himself. He held up a 'Harrods' shopping bag.

'I got you a present today. Open it!' Patrick grinned, handing me over the bag. Inside was a box, and I excitedly tore off the box lid wondering what was inside. Underneath all the rustling white tissue paper, was a beautiful navy gabardine nurse's storm cap lined with a pretty pale blue silk. The exclusive 'Harrods of Knightsbridge' label stitched inside its rim was the icing on the cake.

I tried the hat on, and of course, it was a perfect fit. I was as pleased as punch. This was the best present Patrick had ever bought me, and as it came so unexpectedly, it was even nicer. I threw my arms around him in a 'thank you' embrace, and kissed him on the cheek.

'This is beautiful, thank you so *so* much!' I admired my reflection in Mum's hall mirror. I visualised the SRN badge that would be pinned on the front of it in just over two years time and smiled once again. Now I had the ensemble! I twirled before Patrick posing like a fashion model on a Parisian catwalk. This hat meant more to me than any fur coat ever could.

All in all, I decided it was a very good move for me to go back home. Apart from the travel, there was really only one other disadvantage. At Hammersmith House, there had been a constant and abundant supply of hot water, kept carefully stoked up by the faithful boiler-man. At home, the hot water supply came from an old Ascot geyser. I was so frightened of the 'woof' it made when lit up, fearing it would blow up the house in the process, that Mum always ran my daily bath for me.

However, the bath water went cold quickly, and there was no way of topping it up again with more hot water, so it was very much a quick soak. I ran to my bedroom to dry off after my bath, shivering in front of a small gas fire. It was a very cold house, and what heat the little fire did manage to produce seemed to be sucked straight out of the large sash windows. I quickly clambered into bed, trying to warm up by cuddling up to the Boots hot water bottle that Mum had lovingly placed there earlier. Despite the cold, I was soon fast asleep, not stirring again until Mum brought me a wake up cup of tea at 6pm.

I was lucky that I could sleep so easily, anywhere, anytime. Some of my set could not sleep during the day, no matter how hard they tried or however exhausted they became. They resorted to using sleeping pills, and seemed to continually walk around resembling zombies.

After five consecutive nights of working on a trot, like many of my other colleagues, I'd sleep all day on my day off, get up, get fed and then go back to bed for more even more sleep.

As summer came, it seemed to ram it home that I was missing out on normal teenage life. My skin was pale, unlike the healthy tanned glows of my brothers and sisters. Outside my bedroom window, I could hear the gentle pit and pat of the balls on the tennis court, and the calls of young men and women having fun. Having fun? What was that? I'd rather forgotten what that was.

Most of my spare time was spent sleeping *not* courting, so it is no wonder that Patrick felt he had to make excuses to come and see me whenever he could. He soon realised that around 8.45am each morning, I'd be cycling past Fletcher's the Funeral Parlour on the corner of Brook Green and Shepherds Bush Road on the way home from hospital. On a weekend morning, Patrick's friendly face would be waiting there with a freshly picked posy of flowers. All he wanted to do was go and have a romantic walk in the park with me, and all I wanted to do was to go home and sleep. It was hard for both of us. I don't know who felt worse.

'No Other Love' by Ronnie Hilton was often played on the radio at that time, and I could see Patrick was deep in thought while it played.

'No other love have I

Only my love for you …

Into your arms I'll fly
Locked in your arms I'll stay
Waiting to hear you say
No other love have I
No other love...'

It obviously meant a great deal to him, and I could see Patrick was wishing that I could repeat the words of this song to him and mean them. But the truth is, I could not. My other love was nursing and Patrick knew he had to share me with dozens of other men; namely my patients.

Petrol rationing had ended late that Spring, and things were more or less back to normal. Bob was back to work, and so was London.

Following first nights, our set thinned out even more with first Peggy leaving, then Catherine, Maria and Tania. Catherine gave in her notice after being expected to lay a dead body out of a patient she had nursed. Maria quit after being sent on her own to the Hospital Morgue at 2am to collect a bottle of blood from the blood transfusion store there. Tania could just not cope with the unrelenting regime.

Although we were generally kept to the same ward during a night-duty stint, we were still required to daily check the night-list in case of any changes. Occasionally a very ill patient would require a 'Special', that is a night-nurse whose sole responsibility was looking after that patient. As a result, nurses would be sequestered from less busy departments to cope with any shortfalls.

Sometimes good news would appear on the dreaded notice board, and luckily, I was one of the first to spot it on such a day. 'Six free tickets to The Mousetrap tonight' the notice proclaimed, and I rushed to get my hands on two before someone else grabbed them. Occasional perks such as these were offered out, always at short notice, although Sisters and Staff Nurses

always had first pickings before any notice ever went up for the students to
see.

I took Mum along as a 'thank you' for all that she'd done for me,
knowing how much she enjoyed the Stage too. We had very good seats in
The House that would have normally been very expensive. Patrick felt
jealous, he hadn't seen me for nearly a week and wanted me on that precious
evening off all to himself. I felt caught between a rock and hard place. I
promised to take Patrick the next time, and he thankfully stopped sulking.

I was true to my word, and the next time, Patrick's hopes were high,
as were mine. We were both looking forward to a little kiss and cuddle in the
darkened theatre. It was unfortunate, to say the least, that Sister Shaw had
decided to take some free tickets to that performance too. We had to put up
with her white face glaring at us from just a few seats away.

It was about this time that Patrick decided he wanted me to meet his
parents. They'd been pressing him for some time to take me around, but as
he put it,

'I hardly see her, so I don't see why you should be any different!'

We braved them together one Sunday afternoon. Their lace curtains
twitched as we walked up their carefully tended weed-free path. I wore a
plain blue dress, which tied around my waist to accentuate my feminine
curves, over which I wore a pretty short-cut pearl-buttoned white cardigan. I
completed my outfit with my faux pearl necklace and stud earrings, and
matching white gloves and clutch bag.

'You smell nice!' said Patrick appreciatively. I was wearing my
favourite Coty de Muguet perfume. I was gunning to make the best possible
impression on my possible future in-laws.

Patrick's parent's living room was fashionably chic. There was a lot
of chintz and frill as was the fashion, and the kitsch Vladimir Tretchikoff

green-faced 'Chinese Girl' painting popular in so many households of the time, hung over their grey marble tiled fireplace.

I sat primly on one of his parent's Parker Knoll armchairs, the headrest of which was covered with an embroidered lace cloth. I felt very self-conscious as I drank the earl-grey tea from a fine china teacup, careful to mind all my p's and q's. It was important to me that Patrick's parents approved of me. I could see by the way Patrick's mother was looking me up and down though that she thought I was beneath her son though. I wondered if it was something to do with my working-class London accent that I was doing my best to disguise.

'So, Cynthia, what do you plan to do after your training?' asked Patrick's mother.

I thought it a strange question. 'Why, nurse of course.'

Patrick's mother sat stony-faced. She obviously did not approve of a young lady having a career. Hers wasn't such a strange question, however; many nurses did go straight from graduation to marriage and thus home-making. In Victorian times, nurse training was seen as good preparation in itself for marriage, and although less prevalent, that archaic attitude was still evident in some parts. I was not planning anything of the sort, however. So *that* was her problem with me! I smiled sweetly at her as Patrick discreetly changed the subject.

'Don't worry, they like you.' Patrick told me after we'd gone. I knew that wasn't completely true. Patrick was now 24, already several years older than the average man entering marriage in 1957. Patrick's parents wanted him to find a nice girl and settle down and have lots of babies *soon*.

As Roman Catholics who didn't believe in any form of contraception apart from the Rhythm Method, babies would inevitably quickly follow marriage. A 'nice girl' for Patrick's parents therefore meant a home-maker, not a career girl like me. Despite their taste for fashionable décor, Patrick's parents were decidedly old fashioned, and agreed wholeheartedly with the Church's recent statement that working mothers were 'the biggest blight on Christian society'.

Patrick's parents tolerated me though, as like Patrick thought (but dared not admit to my face), they thought I would soon give up nursing. Then, when I saw sense, I would be fully embraced by the family as the prodigal future daughter-in-law.

I had other things to worry about though than how much Patrick's Mum liked me. The dreaded State Preliminary Exams loomed over me, and having paid my examination fees, I swotted up on anatomy and physiology. If I failed these exams, I was *out*! To help with revision, one week was spent 'in block' in the Training School. It felt very strange after a hectic year to be back with all the other girls from my PTS. Those who had not yet quit, that is! Although it was a stressful time, it was wonderful to be able to sit down all day instead of rushing like a headless chicken around the wards.

Although I was a student, there was no long stretch of summer vacation to look forward to after exams. I got two weeks, and that was it. Holiday dates were given out and I was allotted the last fortnight in June. I was very glad, as this was my favourite time of year, with birds in full song and bright flowers everywhere.

I determined to get as far away from the hospital as possible, and try to forget about my pending exam results.

'Lu, would you come hitch-hiking with me to the Isle of Wight?' I asked my younger Sister Lucille, who was now 15. 'We can stay at youth hostels.'

In 1957, the world seemed a far safer place, and Mum was happy to let us both go on such an adventure. Cars were back on the road in full force, and Britons wanted to seize the motor touring opportunities they'd been denied for so long during the Suez petrol crisis. We explored the Isle of Wight's sites, touring in Morris Minors, Austin Healy's, Triumph Heralds and Ford Anglias. We had a glorious time, and I returned to the hospital tanned and refreshed. It also worked out a cheap holiday.

One really petty hospital rule that really should have been banished years before, was that I had to write and inform Matron *from holiday* that I was returning to duty, Sunday week, as arranged. Her letter went out together with the Technicolor picture postcards of Ventnor and Sandown sent to Patrick, my friends and family. Matron was certainly not getting a pretty postcard from me, and I deliberately used the most plain and boring stationery I had in my possession.

I didn't want to come back to London, but the thought of Patrick's open arms waiting for me at the other end helped take the sting away. That, and my eagerness to know my exam results.

On the 20th July 1957, two days before my first year exam results were published, the Prime Minister, Harold Macmillan said in a speech that was to become famous,

'Go around the country … and you will see a state of prosperity such as we have never had in my lifetime, nor indeed in the history of this country… Indeed let us be frank about it; most of our people have never had it so good.'

'Yeah, right!' I muttered under my breath, as I snagged my last pair of nurse's hose. 'Not for the nurses, though, eh, Harold?'

A few months after Macmillan's speech, in October 1957, The House of Lords talked of finally admitting women to their ranks.

'Maybe the Women Law Lords will do something for the nurses,' said Shirley hopefully.

'Don't count on it.' laughed Claire, who was never one to mince her words, 'Those snobs just look after their own.' And she was right, unfortunately.

Those who passed the first year exams were summoned to Matron's Office. I was luckily one of them, as were Claire, Shirley and Trudy. Sadly, two from my set failed and were unceremoniously booted out. I felt very sorry for these girls who'd put up with so much flack over the year for nothing.

The last time I had been to Matron Godden's office, I'd been trembling like a leaf, clutching a kidney dish containing twelve broken glass thermometers. Today, although still shaking with nerves, I had a happy reason to be there.

With great ceremony, the made-to-measure grey Petersham belt with my name on it, was placed over my grey dress with a smile, firm handshake and warm congratulations. This was the first time I had ever seen Matron smile. I was now officially a 'Grey Belt' or Second Year Nurse.

CHAPTER IX
Grey Becomes Blue

As a Second Year student, I rotated between the various Hammersmith wards gaining the necessary variety of experience. As change lists were posted up every eight to twelve weeks, so different experience was gained, and the numerous procedures were learnt. I carried around my practical training book from ward to ward, which had a list of procedures from the more unsavoury, such as inserting rectal suppositories or observing sputum, to the more pleasant tasks such as feeding a baby. It was each Ward Sister's job to sign this book as I became proficient in each task.

I left home each morning at 6.40am, and after parking up my bike headed straight to the changing room. This was designed for non-residents such as I, and contained our individual laundry boxes full of starched aprons, clean white hats and spare dresses. On exchange of my prized gabardine outdoor hat and coat, Florrie, the always smiling domestic assistant in charge of the room, handed me my cape. After flinging this on, I rushed straight to the wards.

Asian flu' reached the UK in the summer of 1957, and the hospital beds began to get choked up with its casualties. Some 3,500 people died, and the government issued a flu vaccine to those most at risk, including medical staff. I was one of the long line of nurses who stood waiting patiently to be jabbed.

Orthopaedics Ward was packed to the brim with patients with legs suspended in traction, and covered in Plaster of Paris. This ward required constant bottles and beeps because of the enforced bed rest. Most patients were young men, victims of motor cycle crashes or sports' injuries.

The men were bored as they felt fine, apart from being immobile, and they would put their time to ill-use by concocting up good-natured tricks to play on the nurses. One of their jokes was filling a bottle with Lucozade instead of urine, so when the unsuspecting nurse noticed raised sugar levels during a routine test, she thought her patient had suddenly developed diabetes!

The men were very cheeky, and would love to make young nurses blush with their sauciness. As most of us were *very* sexually inexperienced, we were easy pickings.

The ward also had its perks for some nurses. If you were going to find romance in the hospital, it was more likely to happen here. 'After two days in hospital, I took a turn for the nurse!' was a little comic sketch pictured on the front of saucy seaside postcards, and it was so often true.

Many an infatuated young man declared his ardent love for a nurse. Although flattering, most of us realised it was a classic case of 'transference', the men projecting their feelings of gratitude from the nursing care and attention received, and confusing it with love. Most of the men would get over their feelings pretty quickly on leaving the hospital.

'DEAR Jane! Dear winsome Jane!
How you stole in the room (where I lay so ill)
In your nurse's cap and linen cuffs,
And took my hand and said with a smile:
"You are not so ill—you'll soon be well."
And how the liquid thought of your eyes
Sank in my eyes like dew that slips
Into the heart of a flower.' *

---
* Paul McNeely, Spoon River Anthology, 1916

Some men, however, were more persistent. One patient would not accept Jenny's firm 'no thanks' to his asking her for a date. He hung around outside the hospital every day for a month, hoping to get a glance of his Jenny, while smothering her with gifts of flowers and chocolates. In those days 'stalking' was not part of the general vocabulary, and this man's behaviour was not viewed as anything sinister. We just saw it as a young man who'd 'got it bad', and ribbed Jenny mercilessly, asking her when the wedding was going to be. The infatuated young man eventually got the message that Jenny was not interested in him, and moved on.

Real love did occasionally pop up its head though. Diana from my PTS set met her future husband on Orthopaedics ward. Staff/Patient romances were frowned upon, but true love would find a way.

Meanwhile, despite his parents' heavy hints to find someone 'better', Patrick and I continued to go 'steady.' He put up with a lot, and my friends and family constantly reminded me of this fact. I know Patrick got frustrated at not being able to take me to the theatre or cinema for special events because of my shifts. When I did see him, I was often so tired that it was hardly 'quality time'. It took the biscuit when I fell asleep in the cinema during a Doris Day film we'd both been looking forward to seeing for a long time.

Mum was continuing to work in the major Elstree, Ealing and Pinewood productions. She'd recently been working as an extra in the story of the fateful maiden voyage of The Titanic, *'A Night to Remember'* with Kenneth Moore. She had a stinking cold after the filming, which she blamed on being kept in the production's huge water tanks for prolonged periods over three days filming. I tried to keep out of Mum's way while she was infectious, as the last thing I wanted was to be sick.

When 'A Night to Remember' was released the following year,

Patrick and I went to watch it at the local Odeon to try and spot Mum in the background scenes.

'There she is! And there she is again!' we giggled over our ice creams. We both thought it was a fantastic film, even the more interesting because it was true. I'd not personally met a Titanic survivor, but I met plenty of people on Geriatrics Ward who remembered the disaster well.

Geriatrics, G1 and G2 Ward, was exceptionally heavy work, and I regularly trotted back and forth to physiotherapy between shifts to soak up treatment from the infrared lamp for my sore back. As ludicrous and non-understandable as it seemed, I refused to give up. Nursing was my life.

It was also hard to watch once bright, vibrant people lose all their faculties before my eyes. One dear woman on Geriatrics Ward, Mrs Jordan, had gone a little dotty with age.

'Quick, Nurse!' Mrs Jordan's neighbour called in horrified tones, as I helped another patient into her dressing gown, 'Mrs Jordan has shit the bed, and is eating the mess!'

Forgetful patients were also known to hide their little 'offerings' in their lockers or all manner of other strange places, and I needed to be ever vigilant of this. At all times, I treated all the patients with respect, and tried to maintain the little dignity they had left.

The nurse's prayer that I'd cut out from 'The Nursing Times' was on my bedroom wall at home, and I looked at this before I went to bed, to help to give me strength and to remind me to be kind and respectful to all.

A Nurse's Prayer by Alwyn M Heal

Lord, give me grace on this and every day
To do my work the best not simplest way
And to remember that in all I do

The very smallest task is seen by you

Grant to me courage, Lord, when things go wrong
To stop and think and not rush blindly on
And the task I'm set may not seem fair
May I remember Thou, who art there

Give me a humble heart that I may know
That things worthwhile, are not just things that show
For though efficiency and skill mean much
The greatest gift of all is the human touch

Fill me with love that I may realise
The suffering or pain that around me lies
And grant each day that I may seek to share
The burdens of the people in my care

Lord, give me strength to help me play my part
To make my work the essence of my heart
And show me patience and true kindness Lord
That I may spread Thy radiance through my word

So when at night I come back to my rest
I pray thee I may feel I've done my best
And Lord at times I know I forget thee
But please forgive and always be with me.'

    The time spent in blanket bathing, provided an opportunity to get to know each patient better, and I heard countless stories of life growing up in the Victorian age. Many of the stories were so sad; with the common theme being of young lives blighted by war.

    'My youngest brother, Fred, never came back from Flanders, and then Julian and Edward my other two brothers died at the Somme.' Miss Rose told me, with tears stinging her eyes at the bitter memory. 'If that wasn't enough, Father and Sissy died in the great influenza epidemic. Mother was heartbroken. I was all she had left.'

One of Miss Rose's few friends over the last decade had been her cherished West Highland Terrier, Tommy, who she'd had to leave when admitted to G2. Her faithful companion now gazed at his mistress from a curled 7 by 6" black and white photo that took pride of place on her hospital locker. Miss Rose regularly cradled this photo, stroking the image and kissing it. Although her body was rapidly failing her, Miss Rose was as bright as a button, and was depressed and lonely on this ward that seemed so cold and clinical to her.

It was known for patients like Miss Rose just to give up, even though there was no clinical reason for their passing. They were simply tired, fed up with life. Miss Rose went quietly in the early hours of one morning with a nurse holding her hand. I was relieved Miss Rose had not been alone at the end.

I cried and cried at Miss Rose's lonely life, but I felt some relief when she left the ward with the mortuary porter and accompanying nurse. At least she was now free from pain and at peace now with her brothers, Father and Sissy.

All in all, I found Geriatrics a sad and depressing place, with a seemingly continual beep round. As a useful distraction from the emotional drain of the ward, I'd go into the nurse's sitting room to try to relax a little. A radio was always on in the background, and when I was lucky enough to get the chance, I loved to listen to the BBC Home Programme.

'It is five minutes to ten. A story, a hymn and a prayer…' The short service inspired many of us, and gave a boost to tired and flagging spirits. It became a cherished ritual, and the familiar signature tune blaring out gave a warm feeling, as if signalling the arrival of a good friend.

The other shows that became firm favourites for us nurses were 'Hancock's Half Hour,' 'Educating Archie' and 'The Goon Show'. Chuckling to myself while I listened, I worked on an embroidered cushion cover that I had called 'The Marsh'. Many a happy moment was spent stitching a myriad of different coloured Clarke's Anchor Threads into making up my 'masterpiece'. I also knitted Patrick a four-ply wool cable-stitch pullover, as was the fashion. He loved it, and would wear it often.

The radio broadcasts reminded us that the world was going through amazing changes. On the 4th October 1957, the Russian satellite 'Sputnik' was the first man-made object ever to leave the Earth's atmosphere. The satellite orbited the earth every hour and a half. The fact that a Russian satellite was flying over the USA seven times a day inevitably caused American jitters. It had been less than a year since the Suez crisis, and the world was right to feel worried. Sputnik's weight also led to speculation that the rocket that launched it into space may be capable of carrying a nuclear weapon from Russia thousands of miles to the West.

A month later, in November, the Russians launched the first ever living creature into space. The dog, Laika, nicknamed 'Mutnik' by the press, was launched aboard Sputnik II on a one-way trip. Laika had been a stray wandering the streets of Moscow when she was captured and prepared for the space mission by the Russians.

Animal welfare organisations in Britain expressed outrage at the Russian's actions. The National Canine Defence League called on all dog lovers to observe a minute's silence every day Laika was in space. She captured the hearts of people around the world as the batteries that operated her life-support system ran down and the air in her space capsule ran out.

The Russians claimed Laika died painlessly about a week into the flight.*
Laika's coffin circled the Earth 2,570 more times before eventually burning
up in the Earth's atmosphere.

The whole incident received a lot of radio air time, and it had us all
hooked in the nurse's sitting room.

'That poor dog,' murmured Trudy, tears stinging her eyes.

'Those flaming Commies,' grimaced Shirley, 'will they stop at
nothing?'

Claire looked up at us steadily, 'Hey, the Yanks are the ones who
started this. This has been going on for years. The Russians are only getting
all this news because the animal got into space, not just *near* space.'

In 1949, The U.S.A. had used captured German V-2 rockets to
launch four monkeys named Albert I, II, III, and IV respectively, into the
atmosphere to see how they would cope with space conditions. All of the
monkeys survived the upward trip, but were killed when parachutes failed to
open and the rocket nose cones impacted the ground.

In 1951, the U.S. Air Force launched the first record breaking animal
flight *near* space, which resulted in a monkey named Yorick and eleven mice
returning back to the earth alive. They reached a height of 45 miles but it
received little press attention as 'space' officially began at 50 miles. **

---

* Forty years after the incident, the Russians revealed Laika actually died
from panic and overheating just a few hours into the flight.
** Many other space experiments involving animals had been carried out
between 1951 and 1957 by both superpowers. Animals tested space suits,
ejection seats, air quality, and the effects of stress and weightlessness on
living organisms amongst other things. At least thirteen subsequent Russian
dogs were launched after Sputnik II. Five of the dogs died in flight. Strelka,
launched aboard Sputnik V in 1960, later gave birth to six puppies, one of
which was given to President John F. Kennedy. In May 1959, The USA was
able to boast that two monkeys had become the first living creatures to
survive a space flight.

'A man will be going up soon.' Claire looked steadily up at us.

'No, never!' we all exclaimed, 'that's many years away. They can't get them back, let alone alive!'

But less than two years before Sputnik 1's launch, the possibility of interplanetary travel was described as 'utter bilge' by Britain's new Astronomer Royal, Professor Richard van der Riet Woolley. Even the astronomers were having to admit they could be wrong.

I was not sorry when the change list pointed me from Geriatrics to Gynae. Geriatrics had been such a depressing place, and I did not fancy spending my second hospital Christmas in such a sad atmosphere.

Gynaecology ward had an excellent Sister who went out of her way to teach and train her charges through observation. I learnt a lot from her, but there were a few things deliberately kept from me and other trainees.

Abortion was illegal, and generally only talked about in hushed tones, but everyone knew it went on. A far greater percentage of women who were admitted to Gynae were in because of complications to do with botched back-street abortions than even the NHS liked to admit. Many of the women who came in for 'D & C's' came in to have the job finished off properly. It was said that more than sixty percent of the women who sought illegal back street abortions were married. I didn't realise any of this then, and took everything that Sister said at face value. As far as I was concerned, they were 'just' women with genealogical problems.

It was while working on Gynae. that I developed a severe case of vaginal thrush. Being none the wiser, I was terrified that I had caught VD from a patient or infected toilet seat. I was so sore, that despite my embarrassment I got examined, and was very relieved to be told that what I had was merely thrush, and that I'd developed it because I was so run down.

Hammersmith did not have a VD clinic. Any patient with symptoms was referred to 'The West London Hospital' seven miles down the road. Yes, the VD clinic happened to be in the same street where I lived! Martha Clinic attended to the women and Luke Clinic to the men. Looking carefully over their shoulders so as not to be detected, fur-coated heavily made-up dolly birds, prim looking housewives, City Gents in bowler hats, bus drivers and even Vicars went through The West London Hospital's doors for the routine shots of penicillin in the backside.

My second hospital Christmas was spent on Gynae. Ward. Once again, I joined the troop of carol singers, and once again, thick smog engulfed the nation. In December 1957, a horrifying rail crash killed 92 passengers in Lewisham, South London. The disaster happened in thick fog when a train went through a red signal and ran into the back of a stationary engine between St John's Wood and Lewisham station. It was a very anxious time for several patients and members of staff at Hammersmith, as they waited to hear news of whether their loved ones were Okay or not.

The rail disaster put rather a downer on the festivities, with many people in subdued spirits. Outside the hospital, Patrick and his parents watched the Queen give her first Christmas television broadcast to the nation. They were lucky they had a Television set. Our family did not, and few people in Mum's street did either.

In January, the change list despatched me to children's ward. Everyone looked forward to working on the Children's ward, and I just cursed my luck I could not have been there a month sooner for Christmas.

There was H1 and H2, or H3 and H4 ward, and it was luck of the draw as to which ward I was assigned to. I was allotted H3 and H4 ward, where Sister was exceptionally strict. She had been at the hospital for many years and was practically part of the furniture. But she certainly knew her stuff, and the children loved her.

It was pathetic to hear the children wail and bawl for their mother when left alone for the first time on the ward, but they quickly adjusted to their new surroundings.

The children's clothes had to be all washed by hand, and umpteen dirty terry-towelling nappies passed through the sluice. My hands became extra red and sore with the additional wash loads. Preparing my hands with glycerine and sugar was meant to help soothe the redness, but it never seemed to help me.

Bottle-feeding the babies was a much-cherished job, and also meant I could take the weight off my feet for a few minutes while I fed and fussed the ward's newest arrivals.

As Hammersmith was a pioneering teaching hospital, heart operations on 'blue babies', those babies born with heart defects, were performed, and although the technology was still in its infancy, many of these babies miraculously survived.

Despite the surgeon's utmost care, inevitably some tiny hearts could not cope with the stress of surgery. How the ward staff wept, when we were grimly told that baby Johnson or Baby Dixon would not be returning to the ward after all. Although death and dying was part of the daily routine, and something we should have become accustomed to, it took the most hardened nurse not to weep at the death of a child.

The end of year exam once again loomed, with revision time on surgical nursing in study block beforehand. A nice 'rest' in block study was in store. In February 1958, ever thinning numbers from our set met up to cram as much as possible into our exhausted heads. The Surgical men albeit good at their work, were rarely any good at delivering interesting lectures.

In the meantime, Patrick introduced me further to the joys of classical music, frequently arriving on one of our dates with a present of a

78-rpm black vinyl disc that he'd brought me from the HMV store in Oxford Street.

Beethoven, Mozart and Handel became my companions, and joined my collection of big band swing music at home. I found the soothing music helped me relax and de-stress from the pressure of impending exams. In March, many of the nurses, including Janet, had long faces. My younger sisters, Lucille and Diana also looked rather tearful. Their hero, the 'dishy' Elvis Presley, had left them, being forced to report for U.S. military service, as number 53310761 in its ranks.

In May, I was very relieved I was no longer dependant on public transport, as the bus drivers went on a five-week strike. Seven thousand red London buses were off the streets, and the capital was brought to a virtual standstill by cars clogging up the roads in their stead. If I hadn't had my trusty bike, I don't know what I would have done - I would certainly have found exam time far more stressful because of it, that's for sure.

Although trembling like a leaf, I was glad to get exams out of the way. After sitting my exams, a fortnight's holiday wonderfully beckoned. Once again, my sister Lucille and I went hitchhiking, this time around Devon and Cornwall.

Away from London, the roads were quieter, and everything seemed to go at a slower pace. Folk ambled along like they had all the time in the world, picnicking at the sides of roads or at little cafes instead of stopping at huge impersonal Motorway Service stations.

The roads were not only quieter but they were also smaller. Motorways were still a novelty. The first stretch of motorway, the Preston By-pass, inspired by Hitler's Autobahn, had only just opened the previous December. So many motorists went for sight-seeing drives along this novelty on the first day that a queue of vehicles one and a half miles long formed.

The sunshine, birdsong, wide-open spaces, and fragrant blooms of the West Country's Wisteria around the youth hostels made a marked contrast to the stench of London's hospital corridors. It was a different world, and it felt good.

Lu, although younger, was already earning *far* more than me in an office, and had every evening free. As Lucille and I happily munched on our ice-cream cornets on the beach at Penzance, Lu turned to me, the wind ruffling through her long blonde hair. She looked me straight in the eye, and said,

'Cynthia, are you sure you're doing the right thing carrying on nursing? It's been all slog, and what do you get from it? You're constantly exhausted, in pain and broke. Patrick never sees you. You can't afford nice clothes and make-up. Nobody would think the worst of you if you dropped out now, and there's plenty of good jobs you could go to now with your two years training.'

I earnestly gazed back at her, and replied vehemently,

'I will blooming well do this if it kills me! I've come this far. Nobody is going to take nursing from me.' No-one but a nurse could possibly understand my madness, and it was no wonder that Lu looked at me strangely.

It was wonderful to go to the sewing room some weeks later to be measured up for the bright blue petersham belt, which signalled my graduation to third year student nurse status. It was also a sign that boldly shouted to the patients,

'Do *not* ask me for a bedpan or bottle. I'm too sophisticated for that dirty work now!' The patients were so well trained that they would rather burst than break the 'rules'. I really now was on my way.

Chapter X

'Crash, Bang, Wallop!'

'Crash, bang, wallop!' a pile of metal cascaded to the floor.

'Really, Nurse!' yelled the infuriated Sister on Renal ward to the new PTS trainee, 'You must learn to be more careful and quiet otherwise you *must* leave the ward. The sick patients cannot tolerate such noise.' Sister's lips pursed tightly together, and with a grimace, Sister turned to resume her conversation with Professor Morris.

The raw junior, her starched hat all skew-whiff, and her face scarlet, looked as if she wished the floor would swallow her up. She scuttled to pick up the three heavy stainless steel upturned bedpans, and clear up the strewn contents, as the bed-bound audience tittered at the free entertainment.

Now a blue belt, the training had toughened me, and implanted some confidence, and I was able to help the new girls fresh from PTS. I had firmly resolved not to become a third year bully. There were a few from my set who had already let their newfound power go straight to their heads though. There always were.

'Don't worry about Sister. Her bark is worse than her bite,' I winked at the trembling trainee, remembering all too well how I'd felt on my first ward; petrified and all fingers and thumbs. The PTS girl, grateful for some encouragement instead of harsh words, relaxed a little.

'In one of those bedpans was a specimen I needed to test for Sister.' she confided to me in a hushed whisper.

'Well, your patient will just have to produce another specimen for you...' I grinned, 'Easily done!'

As a Blue Belt, I was given more senior nursing duties, but I was unfortunately not exempt from cleaning duties. Sunday afternoons were always earmarked for extra weekly cleaning tasks. In between the extra scrubbing, I'd ferry visitors to bedsides. I'd always feel sorry for the patients with no visitors, and try to stop and have a brief chat with them if only for a minute. It was also known for me to scrounge a bit of fruit or a few flowers off other patients and pass these on to 'the unloved'.

'Nurse, you have no time to waste on idle chatter!' Sister barked, as I tried to cheer-up a depressed looking patient. I hurried off to clean an already immaculately clean cupboard. It didn't make sense to me to be assigned such a fruitless task, when I could be ministering instead in a far more rewarding way to a lonely patient. Still, orders had to be obeyed. The whole ward was scrubbed from top to bottom so that it sparkled even brighter.

Glass thermometers dosed in a liberal amount of carbolic solution stood by each patient's bed, and needed to be taken away and cleaned. Cotton facemasks were rolled up in a special way and put into the mask jar. Many a disgusted face hid behind such these masks; for instance while watching their first ileostomy or colostomy dressings.

After renal ward, I was assigned back to C6, the female surgical that I'd volunteered on as a SJAB cadet some years before. I was put on nightshift. It was too bad that it was during the autumn months when the shortening evenings and later mornings made nights feel very long indeed. However, I considered myself very lucky to have Nurse Morgan as my junior.[*] She was inessential for me, in that she brewed particularly good coffee. I wondered what had happened to Mary, the trainee nurse who had

---

[*] After graduating, Nurse Morgan became Sister at the National Heart Hospital.

been stuck in the sluice on the Queen's visit. Nobody on C6 knew where she'd gone; wherever Mary was, I hoped that she'd passed her SRN exams with flying colours.

As a Blue Belt, the keys to the 'Dangerous Drugs Cupboard' along with other keys were pinned to my uniform dress, and they caused a slight jingle of authority as I walked along.

Every morning, on the handover of shifts, I gave the Night Nurse's Report to Sister, and found it very rewarding to be listened to with respect instead of indifference. I had come a long way in two and three quarter years.

Nurse Morgan had gone to dinner, and as I sat at my night nurse's desk, I stared bleary eyed at my report. My eyelids felt very heavy. All was quiet, save the odd patient muttering in her sleep, and the occasional cough. The ward telephone interrupted my thoughts. It was Sister telling me to prepare a bed for an emergency admission. So it was not going to be a quiet night, I sighed. I was still not allowed to wear a cardigan, and shivered in the chilly night air.

After I had made the bed up for the new admission, Mrs Derby, a patient, pleaded for a cup of tea. Although it was against the rules, I made her one anyway. I fluffed her pillows, and pulled through her drawer sheet so her bed was cool and refreshing. To me, this was real nursing. Mrs Derby gratefully pressed some a two shilling piece into my hand.

'You know I can't take this, Mrs Derby.' Although I didn't wish to offend her, I *had to* place the money back on her locker.

Still holding my hand, she drifted off to sleep. Mrs Derby died three days later of a pulmonary embolism. I was glad that I'd been able to show this patient some humanity in her last days on earth, and not just followed 'the rules'.

As a whole, my third year's training was very interesting, and part of it was spent spreading my net wider than the Hammersmith Hospital.

My third hospital Christmas was spent on secondment to St Mark's Hospital, City Road. St Mark's was just over a mile from 'The Angel' tube station, Islington, but was not deemed reasonable commuting distance for me, so I was required to 'live in' at St Mark's over that period. If I had had to commute daily, I would have felt very afraid to travel in the annual Christmas smog, especially after previous year's Lewisham rail disaster.

St Mark's specialised in diseases of the rectum and colon. I thought it very handsome, as its Victorian red brick gleamed in the winter sunshine. Its cosy atmosphere with its small wards was very different to Hammersmith, and Hammersmith felt large and lumbering in comparison.

St Mark's physicians and surgeons were renowned worldwide for excellence. Everybody I knew who had gone to St Mark's had excellent things to say about it.

My time there was split equally between day and night duty. On the plus side, the Sisters at St Mark's all seemed to be a lot kinder and gentler. On the negative side, there were no kitchen staff working at night, so an unpalatable cold offering was left for the night-staff. It remained untouched until the next day when it was collected. During the day, it was also difficult to sleep because of the noise of smashing beer bottles emitting from the Guinness factory next door to the Nurses' Home.

Patrick as usual proved an angel; bringing fruit and other treats that helped get me through. If he resented having to spend yet another Christmas without me, or having to traipse all the way across London to see me, he did not show it. It was evident he was beginning to feel a lot more hopeful about our relationship, now that my SRN exam was less than six months away. He tolerated my head stuck in books, as he believed he would finally have me to himself once my training was over.

Although I loved Patrick, I was not ready to 'settle-down' and nest. After all, for the most part, a career girl in the 1950s only worked until she was married. I could not have 'it all', and I was not ready to throw my career away just yet. However much I may have stated this, I'm not sure that Patrick really *knew* or understood it.

Patrick thought, hoped and prayed that once I qualified I would feel differently. As time wore on, my career ambition was the cause of increasing friction between us. We'd never argued before, but now it seemed we were falling out over the silliest of things.

St Mark's Hospital was close to Saddlers Wells Theatre, and we were able to attend two memorable performances of the evocative Madame Butterfly, and the beautiful La Boheme. As the stirring Aria rose, Patrick gripped my hand tight, holding onto me for dear life. He knew he was losing his hold on me.

I returned to Hammersmith, and examined the change list. I knew it had been coming, but still dreaded it nonetheless. I was dispatched off to theatre. No-one on my set had a good word to say about Sister Barclay who ruled theatre.

'Keep your head down, and keep out of Sister Barclay's way,' came the consistent advice, as sympathetic hands patted me on the shoulder.

Theatre Superintendent Turner was also notorious for her brutality. Lashing out at juniors, she was unfettered by rules to protect nurses from bullies. She was a sadist, delighting in tormenting young nurses. I would have been a fool to quit just weeks away from finals because of two women's maliciousness, and they knew it, and seemed to deliberately take advantage of it.

During Surgical block, I was invited to join the Royal College of Nursing (RCN), which I did, albeit with some bad feeling. There was a lot of resentment as the RCN at that time did little to complain about nurse's bad pay or working conditions. Nurses were expected to be lady-like and accept their lot as a vocational calling; in other words, be doormats.

I was assigned to F Theatre for my first week. It was badly ventilated and stunk of anaesthetic gases, stale air and sweaty rubber boots. With its minor procedures such as tonsillectomies and circumcisions, F was not the bloodbath of the main D theatre. Sluicing was minimal compared to there. But instruments still needed to be scrubbed and sterilised, rubber boots needed washed down and cleaned, and drums needed packed with dressings, gowns, gloves, swabs and facemasks.

Everything needed to be checked with a toothcomb. Rubber gloves were blown up to check for holes, then powdered and sized before being carefully packed. Facemasks were examined to ensure all tapes were complete before being rolled up and packed into glistening stainless steel drums. The list of duties, as ever, seemed endless, with scrubbing and more scrubbing the order of the day. All the dirty linen needed to be counted and labelled before going to laundry and all trolley wheels were scrubbed until they sparkled, to ensure cross-infection did not occur. Three years training had luckily made me a very quick pair of hands.

Thankfully, F Theatre's Staff Nurse was very pleasant. She would even say 'please' and 'thank you', which was a totally new experience for me. Finding me a pair of heavy rubber boots, and instructing me to don a gown, cap and face mask, she led me into theatre to observe my first operation. As I entered theatre, I was already sweating in the stifling heat. I was glad I did not faint on the surgeon's first incision, as many a young nurse did, although I admit I may have swayed a little.

An eight-year old boy covered in green and white sheets laid deeply anaesthetised on the table. I was privileged to be watching the great anaesthetist, Dr Peter McCormick*, at work. Not for one moment, did Dr McCormick's eyes leave his precious little charge, as the expired gases filled the air and the Boyles' anaesthetic machine did its job. Operating theatre fatalities were far more common in 1959, and anaesthesia far more dangerous. However, a patient dying on the operating table just 'went to another ward' as far as fellow patients were concerned.

'Theatre' was an excellent name for a place of surgery, as there was just so much daily drama there. The surgeons also were huge drama queens. It was not for me though, as I preferred more personal interaction with the patients.

D Theatre was very different from F Theatre when I eventually moved there a week later. In D Theatre, I was treated like dirt. At least in F theatre I had not had instruments and bloody swabs thrown at me by surly surgeons, or been ordered to dispose of newly removed anatomical parts. Luckily, I was spared the horror of taking an amputated leg all the way to the Path Lab. Shirley, was not so lucky, and was physically sick on the way back from her grisly delivery.

However dirty my tasks, it was fascinating to watch the skilled surgeons at work. I was in awe at what they could do. The team of Heart Specialists at Hammersmith Hospital became famous for their pioneering transplant work. That year, they aimed to create anatomical banks for human spare parts, with the hope of repairing or replacing patient's diseased organs. Their new techniques involved modifications of the heart-lung machine invented by Dr. Denis Melrose, enabling the surgeon to operate on a stilled and bloodless organ while the machine took over the patient's heart's function. It was a quite staggering concept.

---

* I later learned that this great man died in his early fifties from a minor infection, leaving a widow and young family. He was well loved at the Hospital by staff and patients alike.

Most of the time at theatre is remembered as mopping and scrubbing bloodstains, and 'keeping my head down'. I was very relieved when my stint in theatre was finished, and I was able to get a placement at another hospital for a short time.

In early March 1959, I opted to spend two weeks at the Holloway Sanatorium, a very large Mental Institution in Surrey. Care of the mentally ill in the 1950s had not significantly altered since Victorian times, and I was left feeling very troubled at watching forced ECT treatments and such-like. The violence and disrespect to the patients was sickening, and I hated the sight of the padded cells and straight jackets. However, Holloway Sanatorium was no worse than any other Mental Hospital of its day. In fact, it had a reputation as one of the best.

The continuous screams and banging from the locked wards haunted me for a long time afterwards. I didn't know how any nurse could stand working there for long. Perhaps the government thought that the £20 a year extra annual salary would tempt nurses away from working in the General Hospitals.

I returned to Hammersmith where the change list directed me to my last ever department of my SRN training, Casualty and Out Patients Department (OPD). Thankfully, I was now back on dayshift, although the fresh spring air could not be revelled in, as my head was stuck in textbooks every spare minute, preparing for my finals.

'You'll like casualty,' said Theresa from my set, in her lilting Irish accent. She had just completed her stint there. 'But,' Theresa warned, 'In OPD they just you to shift furniture about. You'll be well qualified to work for Pickfords Removal Company at the end of it, to be sure!'

Casualty was bright and airy, as the door was always open for the ambulance drivers to stretcher in the latest cases, and for the walking wounded to stumble through.

Sister Gent, who ruled the roost in Casualty, was the youngest Sister in Hammersmith Hospital, and probably the most courteous. Now so close to becoming a Staff Nurse myself, I relished the variety of experience gained within the white-tiled walls. It was constant go, with the intercom crackling frequently, calling the Housemen to urgent cases, but I found Casualty very interesting.

Soothing Kaolin poultices were much in demand, and after I'd finished my stint on Casualty, I'd become expert in their application to all parts of the human torso. My skills with a hypodermic needle and other intra-muscular needles also improved with the umpteen penicillin and tetanus shots administered.

All sorts streamed through Casualty's doors, from the very old, to the very young. The local boy's Grammar School, St Clement Danes, contributed more than its fair share of patients, injured during rugby scrums or cricket matches.

On the weekends, young men would be brought in, with blood all over their silk drape jackets. The Teddy Boys Razor Gangs had been clashing again. Usually their wounds were relatively superficial, and after being patched up and sewn up, they were soon dismissed.

Some of the violence was more serious though. I saw one gunshot wound, and there were whispers it was caused by underworld gangland violence. Most of us would never know who was actually responsible, but the notorious Kray Twins had already established a reputation for themselves as 'hard men', and owned the local Regal billiard hall in Bethnal Green. Perhaps they had been involved in the incident.

It was not unusual for a patient to be brought in dead. One haemorrhaging young woman, 'Anna', was rushed in, literally at death's door.

'She's been up to see that woman in White City,' nodded the porter grimly. He'd brought in more former clients of this illegal 'Medicine Woman' than he wanted to remember. This woman, Anna, although bleeding to death had just been dumped out of a moving car outside the hospital's gates, by perpetrators too scared to show their faces.

There were no need for me to ask further questions as to who exactly the woman on the White City Estate was, when a broken knitting needle and a twelve week old foetus were found floating in the blood in the bottom of 'Anna's bedpan.

Despite nine pints of blood, and the surgeon's best efforts, 'Anna' died. Two lives were lost for nothing. I tried to make myself useful making tea for Anna's grieving relatives, while wondering what Sister Gent would tell Anna's mother her cause of death had been.

My eyes were opened to several other things at casualty. One young man was brought in with severe rectal bleeding. An object had been forced up his back passage causing internal injuries. I was clueless as to how he'd got into such a situation. One of the girls filled me in later at tea-break.

'He's a poof, ain't he?' stated Brenda crudely.

I still didn't really have a clue what Brenda was talking about. Homosexuality, even between consenting adults, was still illegal, and rarely eluded to even in crude jokes. Brenda then graphically described what 'poofs' did, and I went quite white.

'Oh, I see.' I said quietly. I'd never thought before of what homosexuals got up to. I barely knew what heterosexuals got up to. I wondered how Brenda knew.

At mealtimes, our set spurred one another on, as we debated what we were going to do after qualifying, *if* we qualified. Our set would soon be scattered about the country. The last thing I wanted to do after three years slog was more training, but to get a good post in nursing it was necessary to have a midwifery qualification under my belt, even if I had no intention of working with mothers and babies. Like it or not, more training loomed, and application forms and references were sent off to the various teaching hospitals.

Midwifery training was broken into two blocks of six months each, known as Part I and Part II. Passing Part I (The Central Midwives board Part I) was necessary to get a good posting as a Ward Sister, but to get the magical State Certified Midwife (SCM) certificate, it was necessary to complete both parts. Passing Part II opened doors to working in maternity hospitals and on the 'district'.

'I had a reply from Queen Charlotte's today. I'm in, to start the end of September.' said little blonde Joan from my set. I crossed my fingers, hoping that my letter of acceptance would be waiting for me at home. I had also applied to Queen Charlottes Hospital. It was the local choice, but it also happened to be the most famous maternity teaching hospital in England. I was ecstatic when I was accepted to start with Joan in September, pending my SRN results.

Patrick was not happy at all about my decision. He'd become more and more moody and distant. One evening, just after my 21st birthday, he was waiting for me outside work with a huge bouquet of flowers.

'These are for you, darling.' He then fumbled in his jacket pocket. I sensed what was coming.

'We've been going out for three years now. Let's get married.' Patrick produced a gorgeous diamond ring, which was set in a plush velvet-covered box from the jewellers where he worked.

I wanted to throw my arms around him and yell, 'Of course I'll marry you.' My heart wanted to boast, as I proudly waved about the sparkle on my ring finger, 'Look! I really am Patrick's girl!' But I could not. Neither of us believed in long engagements. If I accepted his proposal, it would mean a wedding straight after my SRN, and it would mean me not going onto midwifery training.

'I'm sorry, I can't.' I gulped.

Patrick looked stunned. He turned his face from me, so that I could not see the tears well up in his eyes.

'Maybe in a year or two…' I began.

Patrick sighed heavily a few times.

'Cynthia, I can't wait any longer.' Patrick had had enough.

'I'm sorry, Patrick.' I placed my hand gently on his heaving shoulders.

'Don't!' he snapped, 'Leave me alone!' I left him standing at the Hospital gates.

The next evening, Patrick brought around the Kathleen Ferrier record 'What is Life Without Thee,' as a goodbye gift. Ferrier's version of the song from Gluck's Orfeo ed Euridice was a hit record, outselling even Frank Sinatra that year. 'What is life to me without you?' Patrick was saying, 'I can't go on! *Please!'* It was Patrick's last-ditch attempt to get me to change my mind. I didn't.

Patrick couldn't wait, and I couldn't give up nursing. With a heavy heart, I watched him walk out through the door remembering how full of hope both of us had been just a few years before. Still loving him just as much as I ever had, I had to let him go.

Patrick had been a huge part of my life, and now he was gone. I had little time to grieve for him though. Most of my time when not in Casualty was spent with my head stuck in a textbook.

I went around Casualty in a slight daze for a few days, and then forced myself to pull myself together. I had to, exams were just weeks away. I found Minor Operating Theatre fascinating as well as civil, and watched minor broken bones being reset, and boils and abscesses lanced.

I enjoyed setting up the many trays and trolleys needed for the day. Although boring, it gave me time to think. Each trolley was thoroughly scrubbed and cleaned in the Sluice. Clad in white from head to foot, wearing a long gown and facemask, sterile white covers were lifted carefully from a drum using Cheatle forceps, and then placed on the trolley. From the constantly boiling sterilisers, I'd then lift out the bowls and other instruments that were required, and place them on top of the cloth on the trolley. Sterile dressings and cotton wool balls were picked from the drum and duly placed in a bowl, and this was all covered with yet another sterile cloth. With no windows open, for fear of germs, working in the sluice was almost like having a sauna.

With the constant pulling of bed screens up and down around Casualty, my back was giving me gip, despite less heavy lifting. I found swimming a great relief, and for 4d a time went to the local Lime Grove Swimming Pool, an old Victorian Public baths that had cubicles all around the waters edge to get changed in. Although I didn't like taking time away from study, it was a good opportunity for me to unwind, and a way to occupy some of the evenings that would otherwise have been spent moping for Patrick.

All too soon, it was time to leave Casualty for OPD. OPD had rows of benches where patients referred from their family doctors would patiently await their turns to be seen. OPD was very rushed. As Claire and I crudely put it, it was all 'weighs and wees' from the start to the finish of each clinic. The patient was weighed, and their urine specimens were boiled in a test tube held over a Bunsen burner, to test for sugar. Over my time there, I managed to get quite a few small burns on my arm as a consequence.

I was not allowed to talk with the patients, save to call their name in a loud voice to hearken them to their appointments. By the end of each clinic, I was a little hoarse from shouting all the patients' names above the din of the waiting hall.

One unpleasant task we all hated was clearing up the toenail clippings and soiled dressings after the Chiropody clinic. Far be it from me to suggest that the chiropodist clean up his own mess. Ugh! As it was a hot day, the smell was awful.

The worse part of the job was shifting heavy, solid oak furniture around from clinic to clinic. I was given diagrams of the precise layout of each clinic as per each Medical consultant's preference. It didn't sound at all reasonable to be asked to shift furniture several times a day.

'It's not your job to question what to do, or what not to do. You do as I tell you at *once!*' roared the OPD Sister, her face becoming so pale that I thought she would end up in casualty with a heart attack, when I presumed to complain about this routine. Another black mark soiled my copybook, sent up for Matron Godden's perusal.

The only perk of the boring and backbreaking OPD, was every evening off, and two days off together for a nice long weekend.

OPD Senior was glad to see the back of me when my stint in OPD was through; the feeling was mutual.

I looked forward to being reunited with the rest of the PTS for the final block of revision. Examination fees were collected and paid for, and if successfully passed, more money would be extracted to get my name on the actual State Register.

I had two lots of finals. The In-House Hospital Finals, involving written and practical work, had to be passed in order to sit the SRN. I passed, and was awarded a Hospital Badge and certificate. I then sat my SRN finals. Now followed a six-week period of anxiety awaiting the results.

I chose to work on at Hammersmith over the summer, rather than temp with an agency like many of the other girls from my set had decided. Matron had filled in my reference for Queen Charlottes, and my punishment for choosing to leave Hammersmith was yet another set of nights. I naively thought that I'd seen the back of them. However, I bided my time on Cardiac Ward, intent on earning as much as I could over the summer for the necessary textbooks for Queen Charlotte's Midwifery Training.

One balmy summer afternoon, fierce knocking awoke my deep sleep at home. Because of all the commotion, I sleepily went downstairs to see what all the fuss was about.

Mum stood deathly still clutching a telegram. Mum's tear-stained face was white as a sheet.

'It's John,' she whispered. 'He's dead.'

My brother, John, aged 19, had been working as a Royal Navy Apprentice down in Gosport, Hampshire. Now, the telegram brutally informed us, he'd been brought in dead to Aldershot Military Hospital at 11.02am that same morning. A stolen car had crashed into John's motorbike, and he'd died on impact. I sobbed and sobbed. John had been travelling home to see us for the weekend.

John had been mad keen on boats ever since he was a little boy. One of the first photographs Mum had of John was of a curly haired toddler dressed in a sailor suit. Painted wooden models of navy frigates and destroyers that John had made stood pride of place on Mum's shelves. John, like me, had been following his life-long dream, doing what he loved.

John's last words in his final letter to Mum had been, 'I hope Cynthia passes her SRN.' Now I *had to* pass, for John's sake.

I was devastated at John's death, and really wished I had Patrick's comforting arms holding me close as I grieved. Instead, I and my family clung to each other over those days and weeks, and I worked in a semi-daze as one shift of night duty melted into another at Hammersmith.

The morning of the SRN results, I waited anxiously for the letters to be posted through the pigeonholes in the Nurses Home. I couldn't disappoint John. If I had a thin envelope, it meant a pass, if I had a thick envelope, it meant a fail, as re-entry papers would be included in the envelope. Luckily, mine was a thin brown envelope.

I phoned Mum right away to tell her the good news.

'Well done, Cynth. I knew you could do it. We all did.' Although she never actually said it, I knew Mum thought I was mad for letting Patrick go. And so did I, on many a lonely night. Now, at least, I had something to show for it.

As soon as I arrived home, Mum rushed to bring out the special Victoria Sandwich iced cake she'd made for the occasion.

'Congratulations, Cynth!' she kissed me on the cheek.

Ginger purred contently, as if to say, 'I always thought you'd do well.' The little liar! He thought I wouldn't stick it. Well, I had stuck it, and achieved my SRN, so there, Ginger! Now, I just had to get through my 'midder'.

CHAPTER XI
Stork Duty

I was lucky to get into Queen Charlottes to do my 'Midder' training, as competition was fierce for places. In September 1959, I stepped through its doors, along with little blonde Joan from my Hammersmith PTS set, to start six months training as a pupil midwife.

I started my 'Midder' on the same day that a massive Russian rocket, Lunik II, hit the moon - the first craft from earth to do so. The Soviet Union issued a statement, denying they'd be making any territorial claim on the moon as a result of their Lunik II landing.

'Why not? They're taking everywhere else,' grimaced Joan.

Six well-worn purple dresses and fourteen stiff white aprons were dutifully handed to me by Home Sister as I checked in. Each Wednesday, I was informed, I'd be given a clean white cap. Over my purple dress, I proudly wore my SRN black belt, fastened with a gorgeous silver belt buckle that Anne, my best friend from school, gave me on graduation. She had also passed her SRN, and I was proud of her.

I chose to live at home for my Queen Charlottes training. It was no further than Hammersmith Hospital to commute to, and it would be cheaper. More importantly, Mum and my family still needed me. I also needed them. Despite the flurry of activity about me, it was a very lonely, empty time without John and Patrick in my life.

'Lottie' training was interesting, but tough going. I *officially* worked a 96 hour fortnight, but there were also lectures, studying, and other extra-curricular tasks to do all in 'off duty' hours. After a knackering night duty, I'd be expected to be in lectures at 9am that same morning. Sister Tutor signed my attendance book, so there was no escaping. At least it wasn't recorded in the books whether I actually fell asleep in these obligatory lectures.

As I struggled to keep my eyes open, Nursing Tutors scrawled long detailed notes on the anatomy and physiology of the female pelvis, pre-eclamptic toxaemia, puerperal sepsis and the like on the large blackboard. During practical demonstrations, a foetal doll that was the ugliest child I'd ever seen was put though a model pelvis so we learned the mechanism of birth. This 'baby' tried to come out all sorts of ways, the 'normal' way, upside down, back-to-front, and sideways.

Two weeks into my training at Queen Charlottes, I received a 'royal summons' from Matron Godden, inviting me back to Hammersmith Hospital for their annual Prize Giving. Medals and prizes were to be awarded for the best nurses of my year, judged out of three PTS school sets totalling ninety-one student nurses. I was instructed to wear white gloves, along with the blue Staff Nurse's uniform dress specially run up for me by Hammersmith's hard-working sewing room ladies.

I had mixed feelings on returning to Hammersmith Hospital on the 29th September 1959. On the one hand, I wanted to catch up with everybody, and of course, see who had won the prizes, but on the other hand, I didn't want anything more to do with the place: I had moved on.

Nearly all the freshly qualified girls from my PTS set, along with the girls from the two other sets of 1956 came, some travelling long distances to be there. Two girls came all the way down from the acclaimed Simpson's maternity hospital in Edinburgh. Other girls had just walked across the yard, as they were happily staffing at Hammersmith.

Lots of chatter ensued, as I caught up with everyone's news. Twenty-five out of forty-seven girls had survived the three-year ordeal to become qualified State Registered Nurses. Teenagers had become women. Faces and bodies had matured, and characters had been moulded. We were all changed people.

A significant percentage of girls had got married over the summer, and wore their trophy husbands upon their arms. As I looked at the newly-weds' glowing faces, I felt a pang of longing, as I realised that I, too, could be married by now. I allowed myself to daydream for a minute, imagining Patrick's twinkling blue eyes proclaiming that he was the proudest man there.

Questions were inevitably asked about where my handsome Patrick was, and I sadly had to explain.

'He made me choose between him and midder.'

'I know what...or *who* I would have chosen.' giggled Trudy. Her engagement ring worn since the beginning of PTS was now accompanied by a shining gold wedding band. A newly married Gail beamed, showing off her Naval Captain husband on her arm, and her slightly swollen belly. My heart ached as I wished my brother John, in his naval regalia, could be with me today.

Mum and Aunty Brooks dolled up in their Sunday best were my guests, and mingled with the proud husbands, boyfriends and other family members over cucumber sandwiches.

Miss Buchan, the Home Warden, tinkled background music on the grand piano, as the assembled crowd filtered in and took their seats and programmes for the award ceremony.

At just gone half past two, Matron Godden, the Dean, and the various tutors and professors clad in black gowns and mortarboards took their perches on the platform, alongside the Ward Sisters. Even though today was such a happy occasion, some of these Sisters still could not find it in themselves to smile. One scowled from the platform, so much so, that even Mum and Auntie Brooks commentated on it.

At 2.45pm, sharp, a beaming Matron, in her finest frilly lace cap, her RCN President's medal dangling on a heavy chain as she spoke, gave an introductory pep talk. The Dean then said a few words, and then came the moment we were all waiting for. Right Hon. Lord Colerane stepped forward to present the year's prizes.

More than once I had questioned the system, and was sure I had scored black marks against my name because of this. So much depended on ward reports, and a biased Sister could easily sway the jury. However, my attitude had not prevented me from winning the Distinction award *and* the Pharmacology award.

As claps willed me up to the platform, I recalled the three years of hard slog and heartbreak, and the patients and staff that had brought me this far. Mum looked on, tears in her eyes. She had seen me hobbling about the house after a shift with back pain so severe that I could hardly walk. I received a firm congratulatory handshake from the platform cast, and a prize in the shape of a book. I chose a leather-bound 'Oxford Book of English Verse' for my Distinction prize, and 'A Field Guide to British Birds' as my Pharmacology prize.

After the annual prizes had been presented, the certificates and badges were handed out to all those who'd passed the Hospital finals. Individually inscribed silver hospital badges made by Spink of London, and certificates rolled in a red cylinder-shaped box, were presented to us one by one, in alphabetical order.

I watched the rest of my set collect their badges, Sheila, Trudy, Claire, Joan, and all the others. I remembered the ones who hadn't made it, amongst them, Janet, Margaret and Peggy. The final name was called, and then Miss Buchan started to play a rousing version of 'Jerusalem' on her piano. We stood and sang the hymn with great feeling as the sun streamed through the windows.

As we got up to leave, a photographer motioned for all of us to pose for a panoramic photo. The set of '56 then dispersed, each of us going our separate ways.

'Bye, Sheila! Best of luck for the rest of your midder!' I called, as Mum, Auntie Brookes and I headed off to catch the Number 72 bus home. On the way out, we passed a line of PTS girls.

'You poor cows!' I thought.

~ ~ ~ ~ ~ ~ ~ ~ ~ ~ ~

It was perhaps the PTS girls who should have sympathised with me, as the dragon Sisters of Charlottes breathed hotter fire than any of the Hammersmith's dragons. Because I was only there for a short time, and had already endured three years of bullying, they reasoned I would put up with anything that was thrown at me. And by and large, they were right!

I was determined to get through part I at Charlottes, but there was no way that I was going to give these ice queens the pleasure of doing part II of my training with them. While enduring the abuse, I quietly asked around for recommendations as to where to do part II.

In the meantime, lectures, study and work took up the rest of my waking moments. Each pupil midwife was assigned six new mums and babies on each ward. All mum's stayed in bed for three days following birth, with absolutely no getting up allowed. I was thus kept busy with bedpan rounds. In addition, each of the Mum's private areas needed swabbing three times daily, and babies also needed bathed, fed, changed and weighed. On night duty, two pupil midwives were left in a ward of up to thirty hungry babies.

As always, much of my time was spent cleaning, and many hours of my midwife training were spent changing bed cubicle curtains, threading curtain hooks, and rolling up 'Bunnies' maternity pads ready for sterilising.

I'd occasionally flick through a newspaper lying around the ward. 'Lady Chatterley's Lover' six-day long obscenity trial at the Old Bailey grabbed all the headlines that October, and gripped the nation. Of course, nearly everyone wanted to get hold of a copy of the book to see what all the fuss was about. Frankly, I couldn't be bothered, even if I had the time, which I didn't.

At Charlottes' I was also taught the other side of pregnancy, by monitoring Mum's during antenatal clinics. A patient's case history book had to be scrupulously kept throughout the entire pregnancy and birth, and I was shown how to fill in the books and plot all the various figures onto its graphs.

On one of my first antenatal clinics, I was motioned by an unsmiling Sister to place my ear against the top of the silver ear trumpet attached to a mother's swollen belly. For the first time, I heard the rush of baby's heartbeat. It was a wonderful feeling, although I had to keep a lid on the rush of my emotions, as I counted each beat and attempted to calculate the beats per minute.

I was then allowed to measure the Mum's fundal height with the wooden ruler kept in my pocket, alongside my red and blue biros and scissors. Urine was tested, blood pressure monitored, and the abdomen felt to assess baby's position. As I nervously felt around the mother's baby, I felt a sharp complaining kick against my prodding hands.

'Hey! Get off, I was comfy before you started poking about!' said baby. I couldn't help but grin. It was a wonderful feeling.

From time to time, the phone rang, summoning us pupil midwives up to the labour ward to watch a delivery. Labour ward was certainly an eye opener. We stared open-mouthed from behind glass walls. I along with many other students, were shocked as we saw for the first time just how much pain the women went through to push new lives into the world. However, at Queen Charlotte's like all maternity hospitals, we never called it 'pain' but always called it 'contraction'. Perhaps they thought the name change would make it hurt less.

Baby Thomas, the first baby I watched being born, was thankfully a straightforward delivery, and I blinked back tears as this tiny human took his first breath of air.

Other births I watched were not always quite as straightforward. Forceps deliveries were very messy, and often required the mother to have a subsequent blood transfusion. Forceps babies, their heads battered and bruised, with forceps marks denting their tiny faces had to be cot-nursed for three days. It was painful to watch, and painful to nurse these poor little mites.

'But at least they have come out and been born. They are safe.' grinned Meryl, a beautiful, dark-skinned student midwife from Jamaica, when she saw how upset I was.

Some babies were born with syphilis. They were born with serious health problems including skin sores, a very runny bloody nose, slimy patches in their mouths, inflamed arms and legs, swollen livers, anaemia, jaundice, pneumonia, and sometimes a small under-sized head. About 12% of infected newborns died from the disease. I saw one syphilis baby during my training. It was hard to watch this babe suffer for something that was not her fault.

I had to witness twelve deliveries before I was allowed to deliver a baby with a qualified Midwife's hands guiding me. Every birth was an exciting miracle. This one felt particularly sacred, as with Sister's help, I very nervously guided baby Abigail into the world, on the eve of a new decade.

I wondered what the 1960's would hold for Abigail, and said a little prayer for her as I held her up for the first time. None of us, not even my fellow student Meryl from Jamaica, who claimed to be psychic, foresaw the decade of amazing change that lay ahead for every member of the western world. Even a fool would not have staked money on a man walking on the moon in the next ten years. It was amazing times indeed.

Speaking of psychic, it was funny what nonsense many of the mothers *and* midwives came out with, regarding superstitions concerning the unborn child. Midwives tended to be a superstitious bunch. One older midwife refused to deliver in a house where there was a cat, as cats were said to 'steal a baby's breath.' However, spiders were lucky, as a spider was said to have weaved a web to hide the baby Jesus from the evil King Herod.

Some of the superstitions were very funny. One of the strangest superstitions I ever heard was that because a man and not a woman had handed the mother a cup of tea after she found out she was expecting, it prophesied that she was going to have ginger twins. The mother believed this adamantly. Unfortunately, I was not at Queen Charlottes long enough to see whether this mum's prediction came true or not!

I walked back from labour suite after delivering Abigail feeling on a real high. Subsequent deliveries left me sometimes with mixed feelings. Birth was usually a joyous occasion, but sometimes my strongest feeling was incredulousness at some of the Sister's cruelty. A young unmarried mum, broken-hearted at being forced to hand over her baby, was at best dealt with in an offhand manner, at worse insulted to her face.

'Perhaps you'll remember to cross your legs in future,' Sister Melrose reprimanded the young mum.

One mum had committed the ultimate sin; she'd not only premarital relations, but she'd had sex with a black man. As the baby's head became visible, Sister Melrose's face had a look of total disgust.

'Well, you obviously can't keep a wog baby.' Meryl looked at Sister Melrose incredulous, but didn't dare say anything. None of us did. We kept quiet as we'd been taught. However, I was determined never to become like any of these bitchy Sisters.

One woman was brought in in labour, after being referred from a casualty department with 'stomach pains'. She really didn't know she was pregnant. Even more naive than my fellow classmates had been at Convent School, she genuinely had no idea of the facts of life or how a baby was conceived. She'd just thought she was getting fat, and hadn't understood that her periods stopping were a sign of pregnancy.

Little was spoken about periods. My mum avoided the facts about 'Auntie' completely. It was, she said, 'nature's way of purifying the body.' I'd been given 'Marjorie May's 12th Birthday' a small booklet produced by Kotex sanitary towel manufacturers. In the booklet Marjorie became unwell for three days, and could not bathe or do anything strenuous. She had to rest. It was still a complete mystery as to why she started to bleed on her twelfth birthday. It all sounded quite frightening!

The British Medical Association had attempted to remedy the British public's lack of sex education by issuing a frank booklet called 'Getting Married'. In the booklet, a Harley Street psychologist discussed amongst other things whether chastity was outmoded. The BMA was forced to withdraw the booklet, after protests from doctors. Several BMA members also resigned from the association in protest at its contents.

'All we did,' said the booklet's editor, Dr Winifred de Kok, 'was to state the facts given in the statistics. We wanted to help all young people, instead of only the good ones.'

And the facts were far less young people were virgins when they wed than society liked to pretend. Inevitably, there were victims; five percent of all babies born were illegitimate. Often it was the 'good girls' who got in trouble, after one mistake. A shotgun wedding would usually ensue, or perhaps a visit to the White City Medicine Woman. Either that or being shamefully 'sent away' to have the baby and then give it up for adoption. An unmarried mother in 1960 was viewed as such a disgrace that the General Nursing Council could strike a nurse off the Register for such a 'sin'.

Fathers were never allowed into the labour room. They were usually more than happy not to have to watch the grisly process, but one keen father wanted to be with his frightened wife as she delivered.

'No, you may not!' snapped Sister.

When he protested by saying there were other people present so why should he not also be there, Sister asked sarcastically, 'And what medical qualification do you have, Sir?'

Toward the end of the six-month training, I was able to watch Caesareans being performed. Although it was a bloody process, it was quite amazing to watch the baby being whipped out so quickly.

One lunchtime, Joan was in tears, playing with the food on her plate.

'What's wrong, Joan? Has that bitch, Sister Melrose, been on at you again?' I asked.

Joan quietly shook her head. Her eyes were red raw with crying.

'Mrs Reed had a pulmonary embolism. I was giving her a blanket bath, and clonk, that was it, she keeled over. I didn't have time to do anything. There was no warning.'

'Poor you, Joan. There's nothing you could have done. You know it's not your fault.' I tried to console her.

Joan bit her lip. 'I know. But that poor baby. And poor Mr Reed.' she started sobbing loudly again.

We had watched Mrs Reed's emergency caesarean operation, from behind the theatre's one-way glass windows just a couple of days earlier. It had seemed to go fine. 25-year-old Mrs Reed had needed a four-pint blood transfusion afterwards, but that was common. She was otherwise healthy, and the last person we'd think would have an embolism. Maternal deaths happened rarely, but they happened, even in the best of maternity hospitals like Charlottes.

'I'm so sorry, Joan.' I hugged her.

As time went on at Queen Charlottes, I realised I was right in not wanting to carry on my training with them. When it came time to sit my Part I exams, I saw that I'd been scheduled to work on labour ward the night before, and was expected to sit the exam at 9am, more or less straight after coming off a twelve hour shift. My protests to Principal Tutor Lawson fell on deaf ears. No one was prepared to budge, no one was interested.

'That is it! As soon as I finish my exams, I'm out of here!' I confided to Meryl and Joan. They too had reservations about doing the rest of their midwifery training at Charlottes, having heard horror stories from the set above us. However, they'd not been brave enough to do anything about it, and were just keeping their heads down and going with the flow. Some other girls thought it better to stick to one place for both parts of Midder for the sake of consistency on their C.V.

'It will soon be over!' Meryl grimaced.

I'd luckily been accepted to do my part II at a small maternity hospital called Thorpe Coombe in Walthamstow, East London, to start that September, pending my Part I results. Thorpe Coombe had come very highly recommended to me, and would enable me to gain invaluable 'district'

138

experience as well. The only drawback was that I would have to wait another few months to start it than I would have at Charlottes, but I could spend that five month period earning some more money so it that wasn't that bad.

True to my word, once my exams had been sat, and my case history books were up to date, I left. As my parting shot, I ensured that Principal Tutor Lawson was made well aware of what I thought of her draconian regulations. I then asked for my Part I badge and certificate to be posted to me. I never wanted to see that lot again.

CHAPTER XII
A Pregnant Pause

I decided to use my five months break between 'Midder' by doing some agency nursing. The London nursing agencies were always advertising for staff, and I thought that the flexible hours that I could do agency nursing would suit me well.

I signed up for the BNA Agency and was asked right away if I'd like to go to work at the very plush and private 'London Clinic' in Baker Street. The London Clinic was famous for all the stars that passed through its doors, and infamous for the list of stars that had died within its four walls. I agreed, thinking it would be interesting to see how the 'other half' lived.

I reported for duty on my first day, wearing my own uniform of a plain white cap and dress, over which I proudly wore my black SRN's belt. Right away, I was discreetly ushered up to the 'female surgical' department. This might as well have been called the cosmetic ward, as most of the women were in for nose jobs, eye bags removal or liposuction.

It was all very plush, and all the patients received the finest pampering that money could buy. Everyone at the London Clinic had a private room where even the cutlery was monogrammed.

Most of the London Clinic's patients were pleasant enough; one very large woman in for liposuction paid me to sleep beside her in her chair for three nights, as she was too frightened to be left alone. I viewed it as money for jam after the constant rush involved in the NHS, and happily obliged.

Some of the patients weren't quite so pleasant, believing because they paid for their treatment that they had a right to speak to me like a servant. I bit my lip and took it; after all, I was used to being treated like a skivvy by now, and the patients' curtness was no worse than the Sisters' or Staff Nurses' at Queen Charlottes.

At least the Staff at the London Clinic were civil to me. One of the staff, Diana, asked me if I wanted to go with her to the huge CND demo organised over the Easter weekend that year. I refused, as I believed CND had communist leanings. My thoughts that CND were financed by the Russians was not just paranoia; at the CND demo at the Albert Memorial in 1958, a group of young men in bowler-hats jived to the 'Red Flag' played on a mouth organ and there were also many prominent socialist CND supporters.

Diana was not 'Red' though – she was just afraid. I was too, but surrounded in a climate of suspicion and terror concerning the Cold War, although I hated nuclear weapons, I felt that Britain had little alternative but to proceed with the Arms' Race. If we gave in, the Russians would overtake us and be able to bully us. I decided to work much of that weekend instead.

On the 18th April 1960, Diana and some of the other nurse colleagues she'd recruited to her cause joined one hundred thousand protestors to march on Whitehall to protest about the Hydrogen Bomb, bringing central London to a standstill. There was a lot of strong feeling - just three years earlier, on Christmas Island, Britain had tested its first H-bomb, five years behind the USA. Although I didn't join them, I, with the whole of London was aware of CND's presence. There was traffic chaos for many hours afterward, and I was significantly delayed in getting home later that night.

Spring turned into summer, and as I continued to work at the London Clinic I treated several famous people. Among the famous patients that I tended to was Joe Loss, the resident bandleader at The Hammersmith Palais. Joe Loss was as kind and gentlemanly in real life as I was led to believe by his public persona, and I was very flattered that he recognised me as one of his dancing regulars.

I loved to go dancing at the Palais on the sprung maple floor, with the large glitter ball refracting light around the room. Joe Loss was extremely popular, and he would often be requested to play his signature tune 'In the Mood' three times or more a night as we all loved it so much. None of the other swing bands who played at the Palais could beat Joe Loss as far as I was concerned.

One British bandleader, Johnny Dankworth, had famously turned-down £10,000 to tour South Africa because of the colour-bar policy operated there.

'I don't want to appear as a hero in any respect, but I feel it is time to make a stand on this colour prejudice,' said Johnny Dankworth. Many other musicians followed suit. However, nobody seemed to see the inconsistency with this stance when our own country's dancehalls operated similar policies every weekend. Many of the protesting musicians played at these same British dancehalls.

For instance, in July 1958, it was reported that more powerful lighting was to be installed in the entrance of The Scala Ballroom, Wolverhampton. An Indian had somehow got in undetected, thereby breaching the ballroom's colour-bar rule. A woman had then complained to the management that she was asked to dance by an Indian. The Scala's management promptly promised to the Press,

'This man will be the last Indian to dance at The Scala.' Nobody in Britain raised an eyebrow at this reported comment. This was 'the way things should be'. The only outcry came from perturbed young ladies who wanted to ensure that management enforced this rule so their Saturday nights weren't 'ruined'. Based on this, I wondered why South Africa was so different for the bandleaders to make a stance about.

It was a pleasure though to treat Joe Loss, and as I waved him off home, I promised,

'I'll see you at the Palais next weekend!'

Other patients at the London Clinic were unfortunately not quite as gentlemanly as Joe Loss though. Several very rich Arab 'gentlemen' called me into their rooms. I came in to find them playing with their penises while waving about wads of notes in their free hands.

'Nursie, Nursie!' they leered. It was obvious even to a naïve convent-educated girl like me what they wanted me to do. I walked out of their rooms in disgust while wondering if any girl had been tempted by the huge sum of money on offer. *Perhaps* the clinic had been 'bought', by allowing these super-rich patients to treat their staff like this, instead of standing up to them and risk losing them as clients.

I refused to treat those men thereafter; nervously confiding in Sister Jenson my reasons. She didn't batter an eyelid; she had obviously heard it all before. Sister was well aware of what these men were up to, but decided to just turn a blind eye to it. Sister Jenson cleared her throat discreetly,

'I'll put you back on female surgical.' I was relieved to be reassigned but at the same time angry that these men weren't reprimanded. At least I didn't have to worry about my copybook being blotted; as as a 'temp' I could afford to take a stand.

The incident left an unpleasant taste in my mouth though, and when my family dentist told me he was looking for a dental nurse over the rest of the summer, I leapt at the chance to work for him.

I worked for him over the remaining six weeks of the summer. After months of working at the patient's bottom end, it was rather strange to now work at the patient's top end. Already, the overstretched NHS had had to introduce prescription charges, and a £1 flat charge was paid for all NHS dental services. I found the dental work very interesting in the short term, although I would not have wanted to remain there long as I'm sure I would have got bored quickly.

In September 1960, my red alarm clock was packed up into my pale green trunk ready for my travels once again. My mother waved me off to start part II of my midwifery training at Thorpe Coombe.

Thorpe Coombe Maternity Hospital had opened in 1934. Its buildings incorporated the mansion in which the famous Octavius Wigram, who'd been on duty with the Westminster Light Horse Brigade, who'd denied Queen Caroline entry to the coronation of her husband, George IV, had lived. The hospital, of some 70 beds, was in the forefront of many developments in midwifery.

London Transport was still working on the 11.5 miles underground line between Victoria and Walthamstow. Started the previous year, it was the first London Underground railway to be built since 1907. Rather than change umpteen buses and then catch the trolleybus to Walthamstow, I chose to splash out on a taxi instead.

Bob's taxi dropped me off at the large shared house at 17, Carrisbrooke Road, E17 that was to become my home for the next six months. This time, I insisted Bob took my fare; I'm sure he still undercharged me though.

I was greeted by the Superintendent, Miss Chadwick, a woman whose smile lit up her whole face. She shook my hand warmly.

'Welcome, Nurse Carstairs. I do hope you will be happy with your time with us here. Let me introduce you to the rest of the girls.' I was quite taken back by Miss Chadwick's warm civil manner.

I discovered that I was part of a small set of four girls. As well as myself, there was Violet from Trinidad, Madge from the West Indies, and

Peggy a fellow Londoner. Superintendent Miss Chadwick, QN was in charge of the house and her girls. A real mother hen, she ensured the house was a warm and friendly place, a home from home coming complete with a cat. I'd struck gold! There were no petty restrictions, with no one having to shinny up the drainpipe to get in after a night out. Boyfriends were welcomed, and given a nice tea rather than icy stares. We each had our own bedrooms, made fresh and homely by Matron Chadwick. If only Joan and Meryl back at Charlottes could see me now, I thought, as I threw myself back onto my cosy bed. There were even some flowers in my room!

Lectures continued at Thorpe Coombe, but far more time was spent on practical experience in the hospital and on the district in the East End. Once again, I'd struck gold; that would mean less time cleaning and doing other mind numbing tasks such as threading hooks through curtains!

Being 'on the district' entailed needing some form of transport. None of us could afford a car, so we resorted to bicycles. Luckily, I was used to cycling, but Madge and Violet were not. In fits of hysterics, I taught them both how to ride a bike. Many wobbles later, they succeeded. I was rightly very proud of my students!

The Cook at 17, Carrisbrooke Road, made some wonderful meals for us hungry students cycling about the district all day.

I was given a district nurse's black bag, a black leather Gladstone bag, containing a metal box covered in serge cloth, complete with contents. Each item, such as trumpet shaped foetal stethoscope, long lengths of rubber tubing, funnelling, catheters, glass thermometers, glass syringes, and rubber gloves were placed in a separate washable white cotton bag within the box. Once a week the black bags were thoroughly cleaned and then polished, the instruments sterilised and placed within fresh clean cotton bags.

This bag perched on my bicycle handlebars, alongside a Gas and Air or Trilene machine. I rode around my district with my apron folded and tucked under my black SRN belt.

Walthamstow had been bombed badly in the war. As well as the dreaded doodlebugs, mortar bombs, and rockets, the Germans had dropped land mines by parachute over the area. Just one of these landmines could have a devastating effect. For instance, a landmine going off at the Bell, Walthamstow, rendered one hundred houses uninhabitable. Amazingly, only one person had been killed by the blast.

As I cycled through the streets of terraced two up and two downs, the testimony of the East End's suffering in the war was still all around me. A row of houses stood, with a gaping hole at the end that had been the unlucky house that had been hit. Children in shoes that had the toes cut off because their parents couldn't afford to buy them new ones, played in their neighbour's backyards, that were bombsites still full of wartime rubble and debris.

Despite their conditions, the people were happy, and there was a strong sense of community. Hitler and his entire arsenal had not managed to destroy the plucky East End Spirit, but The Housing Subsidies Act of 1956 had. Unfortunately, the policy of slum clearance started during the 1950s had a disastrous and irreparable impact on east London, where whole streets were demolished for tower blocks, and communities were divided. In 1960, work was still underway on clearing the bomb-damaged buildings and slums, and in the meantime many of my Walthamstow 'customers' lived in this sense of no man's land.

Although a poor area, Walthamstow had a lovely atmosphere, and I'd often see my 'customers' and their bumps or new babies when I was out and about. Many a time, flowers from grateful mums brightened our living room at Carrisbrooke Road.

I got to know the mums through antenatal visits at Thorpe Coombe Hospital's outpatient clinic, and through visiting Mums in their homes four weeks prior to their due date. I arrived at meticulously scrubbed doorsteps that gleamed in the autumn sun. I'd always be offered a warm Cockney welcome with endless cups of 'char' and plates of homemade fruitcake.

I looked forward to attending my first home birth, and the call finally came in the early hours of one morning.

'Don't worry about bringing a gas and air machine, I already have one. Just bring your bag and yourself!' commanded Sister Marks, a veteran midwife on the district. I jumped onto my bike, flicking on both the lights of my small Ever-Ready bicycle lamps, and cycled off into the night to assist Sister Marks at the patient's home.

Sister Marks showed me the ropes - our instruments were put to the boil straight away on the gas cooker, newspapers were placed on the floor to protect the carpets or floorboards, and the dad was kept busy out of the way making pots of tea. Luckily the birth went well, with no complications, and as I assisted Sister Marks to bring forth the family's fifth child, a little boy, I praised God for another miracle safely delivered into my rubber-gloved hands.

No midwife wanted a birth to go wrong. But there were times when it did. It was inevitable at some point that I'd have to confront a stillbirth.

One day, when I was on labour ward at Thorpe Coombe Hospital, Peggy motioned for me to come quickly to another ward. I was one of the few Roman Catholic members of staff, and was asked to perform a 'baptism' for a little girl who hadn't made it. The baby's battered head hung at a slightly peculiar angle, bruised with red forceps marks, showing the obstetrician had tried his utmost to get this little one out in time. I held this otherwise perfect infant, and offered her up to God's tender mercy. The mother's empty stare and haunted expression as she clutched her dead daughter has haunted me ever since.

My days at Thorpe Coombe were otherwise very happy days. I wished it could go forever, but like everything, I had to move on once I'd passed Part II and got my elusive State Certified Midwife (SCM) qualification.

'What are you going to do next, Cynthia?' asked Matron Chadwick towards the end of my training. There were lots of job opportunities opening up to me now.

'I'm going to be a Queenie!' I replied. I was so impressed by Miss Chadwick and her colleagues, I'd made my mind up to be a Queen's Nursing Sister or Queenie, just like them. Matron Chadwick was touched. She recommended I apply to Kensington District Nurses Association. I valued her opinion, so determined to do so right away.

'And then what will you do after your three months at Kensington?' Matron Chadwick asked softly.

'I'd like to go on and do Health Visitor training at Battersea Tech.' I'd loved being out and about, working 'on the district' at Walthamstow, and the one year's Health Visitor training would open more doors for me to get a good District Nurse's position.

'You should get someone to sponsor you, Cynthia, for your training at Kensington and Battersea. It will help ease the financial burden on you. I suggest asking a Nursing Association in the area where you would eventually really like to work. Where do you want to go?'

I thought for a moment. As much as I loved London, it was so dirty. My face and hair got so filthy cycling every day amongst the car and bus fumes. I longed to be in the fresh air, languishing in the chocolate-box villages that lay at the foot of the gorgeous green Sussex downs.

'Sussex would be wonderful.' I remembered a daytrip that Patrick and I had taken to the Sussex Downs a couple of years before. Patrick had borrowed his father's Triumph Herald, and we'd taken a picnic lunch along with our walking boots. As we lay on a rolling slope near Devil's Dyke, the late afternoon sun beating down upon our faces, Patrick told me he loved me for the first time. It had been a wonderful day. I sighed.

'Yes, Sussex.' I said to Matron Chadwick firmly.

I applied to the East Sussex County Nursing association for a scholarship to sponsor me over the next fifteen months, and received an acceptance letter in due course.

During the last few weeks of my time at Walthamstow, I kept bumping into Charlie, a gas engineer and local councillor, down the local market. Serious, broody, and very good-looking, he looked the business on his moped. Charlie's Buddy Holly style spectacles and his baggy trousers that were slightly flared told me he was obviously a keen follower of fashion.

'What do you reckon to a date then, Nurse Carstairs?' he asked cheekily.

'Ok then, you're on. Pick me up at eight!' I agreed.

I went on a few dates with Charlie. We went to the cinema to watch Ben Hur, and down the local dance hall to jive the night away. Matron Chadwick met him one evening when he picked me up from Carrisbrooke Road. She thought Charlie was a good catch and told me so in no uncertain terms, but now I'd determined to become a Queenie and Health Visitor there was another year and a half of training before I would even consider letting love into my life. I also was very wary of hurting someone as badly as I'd unintentionally hurt Patrick.

Just seven months after we'd broken up, my best friend, Anne, broke the news that Patrick was engaged to someone else. I was shocked. Part of me still held onto the thought that we'd reconcile at some future point. Now my dreams were brutally shattered. We'd no longer dance to 'Some enchanted evening' to Joe Loss's orchestra. We'd no longer lie looking up at the sky on the beautiful Sussex downs. I'd no longer hear those three little words. I choked back my tears.

'He's on the rebound for sure, it can't be love.' Anne reassured me, as she gave me a quick hug. I wasn't sure of anything anymore.

'I hope he's happy.' I whispered. And I meant it.

After six months in the East End, I passed Part II 'midder ', and received my SCM qualification in the spring of 1961.

In April 1961, Soviet cosmonaut Yuri Gagarin became the first man in space, at the same time as I packed my faithful green trunk to go into my own unknown territory. Just a few years before, Gagarin's feat was labelled as impossible by the world, and just a few years before, I'd been given the prognosis by Daddy Wimbush that my back wouldn't let me get this far. Well, I had managed despite all odds. I'd proved the doubters wrong.

I was very sad to leave Walthamstow for pastures new at Kensington District Nurses Association. I gave lots of hugs to Madge, Violet and Peggy, Carrisbrooke Road's resident cat, Cook and of course Matron Chadwick.

'Keep in touch!' she waved. I promised I would, and meant it. Matron Chadwick was to become a very good friend over the years, and many years later sent me a card inscribed to 'the best pupil I ever had at Carrisbrooke.'

Matron Chadwick had inspired me to become a Queenie, and now I was to begin that part of my nursing adventure.

CHAPTER XIII
A Royal Duty

The Queen Victoria Jubilee Institute was founded in 1887, and it was they who set up the Queen's Institute of District Nurses. Queens Nurses were also known as Jubilee Nurses and were often affectionately dubbed 'Queenies'. Well respected around the country, I was about to join a much-loved institution renowned for its excellent nursing standards. My fourteen weeks 'Queenie' training at Kensington District Nurse's Association started in May 1961. As Kensington was the neighbouring borough to Hammersmith, I lived back at home throughout this period.

I was led into the very plush changing room of Boyd Cooper's Nurse's Outfitters shop in the West End. For the second time in my four years of training, I was being measured up for a brand new nurse's uniform.

My Queenie outfit consisted of four pale blue short-sleeved cotton dresses, with six detachable semi-stiff white collars and cuffs. I was also handed over fourteen white cotton aprons. I had to buy the compulsory three pairs of white gloves myself. My outerwear was a smart navy gabardine raincoat. The cap was dark navy serge, rather like a deerstalker in that its flaps could be pulled down over my ears to protect against the elements. There was also a gorgeous plush velour hat that although smart was not practical in the wind and rain. The only thing missing now from my outfit was the silver-braided Queen's Institute of District Nurses Hat Badge, and bronze medal, which I was determined to display on my uniform with pride in the near future.

My Queenie training mainly consisted of practical work, but there were some lectures. I was in a small set of fourteen students. Thankfully, no lectures were given on days off, and even more wonderfully, there was no night duty. I'd struck gold yet again!

The first lecture was given by a Miss Gray, who was the chief superintendent of the Queen's Institute of District Nursing. Miss Gray referred to the many pills a patient had to swallow in their life, but, she looked sternly at us, the bitterest pill of all that the patient had to swallow was old age. She made this into an acronym, and it stuck with me; 'Poverty, Illness, Loneliness, and Loss of friends'.

Most of my patients were elderly and infirm. The Kensington 'diocese' was split into districts, with the Sisters taking the richest areas for themselves. My assigned district was St Quintins, so named after the leafy St Quintin's Avenue that dissected it. It was the furthest North of all the districts, around six miles away, and so would require the most cycling. Still, I was well used to having to cycle miles each day by now.

Kensington was a district of contrasts, from the very rich to the very poor. It was to prove a very different district to Walthamstow. Instead of dirty-faced cockney kids opening the door of a 'two up and two down' and then shouting for their heavily pregnant 'ma', it was not that unusual for a silver-haired butler to discretely usher a Sister into a gleaming hallway of gilt mirrors and Turkish rugs to be seen by 'the lady of the house' . Yardley lavender soap and lace-trimmed hand-towels were politely laid out for Sister's use to wash their hands with.

However, the majority of my patients lived on the Peabody Estate, four groups of three stories high, redbrick Victorian buildings with rounded doorways, bordered by a communal area. They'd been built for London's poor as a direct result of the Peabody Trust set up in 1862 by the American philanthropist George Peabody.

The people living on the Peabody Estate at that time were made up of the poor and desperate, and newly arrived immigrants from the colonies. The estate had something of a reputation for violence, but in my Queenie uniform, I never felt scared. I was greeted with nothing but warm smiles wherever I went.

As I wearily trudged up the steps of the WX block, children crowded around me and fought amongst themselves to be given the honour of carrying my bags, or minding my bike. I never had to fear that my bike or bag would be stolen, despite the fact it was such a poor area.

Harold Macmillan when he'd been re-voted in in 1959 stated that, 'This election has shown that the class war is obsolete'.

To quote 'The Crickets' chart hit, 'That'll be The Day'! Macmillan was either blind or had not ventured far from Westminster. The divide between rich and poor was as obvious as ever.

Each morning, I had to report to 'base' for instructions. As the clock chimed eight, fourteen QN students and eight fully-fledged QN sisters stood quietly in a horseshoe shape in the gleaming room that had once been the drawing room of a smart Georgian Town House. The Superintendent Miss Balfour, and her assistants Miss White and Miss Wood, clad in navy blue dresses, with silver medals dangling from their necks, dispensed instructions and advice along with daily duties from an individual duty book for each area.

Fourteen black leather Gladstone District bags stood unlocked, and packed ready for a speedy getaway in the District Room. The bags stood side by side on pieces of newspaper, the newspaper being placed on the shelves to prevent any bugs jumping inside the bags – not that there was any of course!

Sometimes, along with my daily duties, a bed-bug spray was pressed into my hands, with the command to spray a patient's bed, on the advice of a disgusted QN Sister who had visited the patient the day before.

153

Around 8.20am, rain or snow, we pedalled dutifully off to our various districts, with our faithful District bags perched in the front bicycle baskets, and a satchel strapped on the back carriers. Each patient was instructed to collect soap, towels, pieces of newspaper and other items needed by us into a cardboard box known as the 'nurses box'. Nurses Notes would also be placed in there. However, we couldn't depend on patients providing the correct sanitary items, and so we also had to carry around a small leather satchel containing a hand-towel, soap and nailbrush.

Diabetic patients who were unable to inject themselves, such as Mrs Morris, were my first port of call each morning. Doors were nearly always left open for me; I just knocked and entered. Visiting Mrs Morris brightened my day. She was near blind, and lived in a newly built tower block. I wondered which vibrant East End Community Mrs Morris had been ripped out from.

The first day I'd visited her; I knocked tentatively on her door and called,

'Hello Mrs Morris, I'm your new nurse!'

I then heard a chirpy,

''Allo Nurse!' from her apartment. It wasn't Mrs Morris feeling so chirpy though, it was her pet budgie Percy! As I got up to wash my hands after administering Mrs Morris's insulin injection, I heard a loud, 'Bugger off!' coming from Percy's cage. He certainly didn't mince his words, did that budgie. After a strict telling off from a red-faced Mrs Morris, Percy hid his head in shame. Percy never swore at me on any of my subsequent visits.

Visits to other patients that day entailed changing their dressings, washing and bathing them, shaving them, dressing them, brushing their teeth, changing their beds, delousing their beds (known as bug technique), making tea, letting the dog out for a pee, plus of course ministering essential words of comfort.

My customers although predominantly elderly, were a mixed bunch. I'd cycle from nursing an elderly gentleman with a war injury, to giving an iron shot to an anaemic young mum, to bathing a lady dying from cancer.

At 4.30pm, a similar ritual to the morning one was carried out, where updates and evening duties were fed out from headquarters.

Hospital X-Ray departments sometimes requested I administer a Colonic Lavage to get a patient's bowel clean for a pending x-ray. Bucketfuls of water were needed for this process, it wasn't pleasant for me or the patient, but it was an important part of my job. The only positive thing about the laborious process was that it gave the patient ample time to talk with me about their fears.

After visiting Mrs Morris and her Percy, it became part of my morning routine to give a vaginal douche to a Mrs Schwartz who was slowly dying from cancer of the uterus. This douche gave some pain relief and comfort, and as she slowly drifted off to sleep, Mrs Schwartz demanded that I sit down and have a cup of coffee with her daughter afterwards. I nursed this dear lady until she died, holding her hand as she breathed her last and departed for another world.

Part of my Queenie training involved learning about the various voluntary agencies dedicated to helping the suffering. A young cancer patient, Mrs Webster, on the Peabody Estate, very obviously needed more bed-sheets. I telephoned Marie Curie Society for Cancer Relief to request some financial assistance for Mrs Webster, and was very glad of their no-nohsense approach, with no red tape or committee approval to hurdle through.

'Buy the sheets for Mrs Webster and send us the bill.' said their administrator generously. The Webster family were told they were spare sheets from the Nurse's Home. Later, Marie Curie gave me cash to buy brandy for Mrs Webster too. As her cancer worsened, so my visits to Mrs Webster increased from one visit a day to three. Right at the end of her life, morphine injections needed to be administered at 10pm, and we students all took it in turns to make this nightly visit.

I enjoyed my time at Kensington, and all too soon it was over. Exams were duly sat, and in 'flaming' June, a garden party was held at the Nurses Home, attended by some of the patients. It was a chance for many of us to say goodbye as we headed on to the next phase of our lives.

On successful passing of my exams, I was posted my bronze medal. The monogram to the front of my medal depicted a crown above the letters QV1 and the date 1887. On the rear my name and number from the roll of Queen's nurses was inscribed. I was number 279974, and now a fully-fledged Queens Institute of District Nursing Sister. It was now time for me to leave Kensington.

There were a few weeks left before my Health Visitor Training started at Battersea College of Advanced Technology. It was only fair that I do a little bit in return for my sponsors, East Sussex County Nurses Association. They wanted me to relieve one of the Sisters in Sussex as she took a well-earned fortnight's holiday, and I eagerly agreed. I regarded it as a sort of holiday, as despite the hard work, Sussex's rolling green hills and clean fresh air and birdsong made a welcome change from London's grime and bustle.

The last time I had been in Lewes had been on an Easter 7/6d rail day-out known as a 'British Railways Ramble' with a group of five hundred or so Londoners. We hiked for around a dozen miles across the gorgeous Sussex downs, revelling in the gorgeous crops of daffodils.

Now I was taking the train again to the pretty little town that I'd taken such a shining to on my previous visit.

'This is Lewes; this is Lewes' yelled the railway guard, as carriage doors banged, and steam loudly hissed from the engine. I alighted onto the platform, dragging my trusty green trunk behind me.

I'd been told that someone from Lewes would meet my train, and true to their word, a dark-haired Sister, dressed in her smart blue uniform, waved at me from the other end of the platform. She quickly marched up to me as my train departed with a loud wail, and shrill squeal of the Guard's whistle.

'Hello, I'm Sister Taylor. You must be Sister Carstairs. Welcome to Lewes! Let me help you with that thing!' Before she could reach for my trunk, the porter already had it in his hands.

'Where to, Sister?' he asked, touching the brim of his British Railways Issue Cap.

Sister Taylor led us to her company car, a little Ford Anglia. The porter would not touch the coin tip I pressed into his hand.

'No, Ma'am, I can't take this. Not when you nurses do so much for us. God bless you!'

Her car took us to the rented house that Sister Taylor and the other two sisters shared together on a sprawling council estate. Although this estate was the least attractive part of the town, it was gorgeous compared to the Peabody Estate where I'd been working just months before. Many of the residents had spent a lot of effort into making their gardens pretty, and the last of summer's bloom glistened in the bright Sussex sunlight.

Sister Taylor and her colleagues quickly made me feel at home, and I soon got to find my way around Lewes. Lewes was a beautiful little town, albeit very hilly, and more often than not, I would be pushing, rather than pedalling my bike about its winding streets. I wondered if this was where I would end up working full time after I finished my training at Battersea.

I loved my time at Lewes, and my fortnight's work placement there seemed to be over in the blink of an eye. I'd fallen in love with the town, and was glad that my time there lived up to my expectations. It was hard work, and my legs ached after all the hill climbing on the bike, but I already looked forward to returning there.

Now it was onto Battersea, a totally different kettle of fish.

CHAPTER XIV
Salad Days

My Health Visitor's course at Battersea College of Advanced Technology, London, was a very different experience from the rest of my nursing training. For one full academic year, I wore civvies, and away from hospital starch and discipline, I began to feel human once again. I lived at home and cycled the seven miles to Battersea and back each day.

Despite the travel, I had more leisure time than I'd ever had since eighteen. As one fellow student, Molly, put it,

'Every weekend off, and we can sit on our backsides all day!'

I revelled in my newfound freedom. Long leisurely lunch breaks were spent sitting in the park opposite the tech. soaking up the sun, and I used my evenings to play hockey or tennis. Afterwards, I could take lots of time to get dressed up ready to go out dancing at the Hammersmith Palais. I could even go out on proper dates at 'normal hours' and have 'normal' boyfriends!

Patrick was now married, so I had to move on. I'd bumped into him and his radiant new wife by accident not long after their wedding. She was not at all like me, I noticed. Her long dark hair was brushed into a time-consuming beehive, and she wore an elegant pink twin-set. Her pencil skirt sharply contrasted with my flared skirt. Around her pale throat, hung a string of pearls, bought from Patrick's jewellery store no doubt. The meeting was very awkward, and I think Patrick and I both wished the ground would swallow us up. I made my excuses and rushed off. I was surprised how upset and emotionally churned up I was. Patrick's poor wife was clueless as to my identity. She looked happy, and it was better it stay that way. I couldn't hanker after a married man. Marriage was for life, so that was it. I'd blown my chance.

A stream of eligible suitors came and went through my mother's door, but none of them held a light to Patrick. Still, I tried to forget him; I had to forget him, and forced myself to go out on other dates. Besides, I was still a career girl, I reassured myself. I just wanted to enjoy myself.

I studied health of the schoolchild, health education, public-speaking and how to teach health in clinics that I'd be running in the future. There were lectures also on home-making and economical cookery. We were all expected to buy 'Battersea College of Technology Recipes for Household Cookery' at 2/6d a copy. Weekly exams kept me on my toes, so there was no slacking.

With having extra leisure time, I was able to keep a little bit more abreast of current events. Every time I went into the college refectory, a group of students were having a heated debate about one topical event or other.

One particular group at college seemed to love to sit and debate more than any others. The Beatniks or 'Bohemians', identifiable by their sandals, chunky black sweaters and black berets and dark glasses sat in the corner chain smoking cigarettes while using words like 'hip,' 'cool' and 'groovy.' None of the Beatniks were on my course, they favoured the artier courses, but it was interesting to hear them speak about current events.

The cold war was gaining momentum. Every time I looked in the papers, Khrushchev or the newly appointed youthful president of the United States, John F Kennedy seemed to be having a war of words. I liked Kennedy and his beautiful young wife, Jacqueline. They seemed to be a model couple. I, like most people at the time, believed Kennedy to be a man of high moral character, as he was a committed Roman Catholic. If anyone could bring hope into this bitter cold war, I believed Kennedy could.

On the 13th August 1961, Berliners had awoken to a divided city. Troops in East Germany have sealed the border between East and West Berlin, shutting off the escape route for thousands of people fleeing from East Germany.

Then that October, as if to antagonise and bait the rest of the world, Russia exploded the world's largest ever nuclear device over the Arctic island of Novaya Zemlya. Shockwaves from the explosion were recorded just up the road from Battersea at Kew. Vivid recollections of the nuclear film seen at PTS resurfaced in my mind.

Lord Home, The British Foreign minister, said,

'Eighty-seven nations appealed to the Soviet leaders to spare the world the explosion of the 50-megaton bomb, which endangers the health of many millions of people. The British government share the indignation which will be universally felt at this wanton disregard for the welfare and safety of the human race.'

In the meantime, The United Nations practically begged Russia not to continue with its nuclear testing programme. All I could really do was cross my fingers and pray. It was all beginning to get very scary again. Those who were part of the CND group at Battersea started seeing their numbers swell considerably.

My coursework continued, and as 1961 faded into 1962, I went on a few placements with social workers and public health inspectors, seeing how they worked in the community. One Public Health inspector, eventually married his placement, so there were perks for some of us!

In December 1961, The Health Minister, Enoch Powell, announced that the birth control pill would become freely available on the NHS. We had lots of debate on campus as to the rights and wrongs of the government's decision.

At the time, I didn't even question the Catholic Church's stance on all forms of contraception. The Pope said it was wrong, so as far as I was concerned it was wrong. There was no debate.

'It will empower the women not to having to become slaves by bearing lots and lots of children.' said Molly.

'It will encourage sluts and prostitution.' said Teresa, who was a Roman Catholic like myself.

'It will stop unwanted children being born.' argued Molly.

It was hard to argue with that. Hundreds of children currently filled Dr Barnardos homes, looking to be re-homed. An adoptive couple could by and large take their pick of babies from an orphanage. There were no lengthy waiting lists or extensive social work reports to complete.

'It will stop the back street abortionists.' mused Pat. Surely, it could only be a good thing if the White City Medicine Woman was put out of business.

Abortion was also becoming a hot topic at college, as 'Quality of life' suddenly became an important issue for discussion.

The drug Thalidomide, widely used for morning sickness, was taken off the market in late 1961 after tests revealed it harmed the foetus, causing babies to be born severely handicapped. Public attention was drawn to the quality of life abortion issue by the well-publicised case of an American woman in 1962 who sought to end her thalidomide pregnancy. Sherri Finkbine's request for an abortion was denied by a hospital and a judge in America, and she eventually went to Switzerland to terminate her pregnancy where it was revealed that her aborted baby had been quadriplegic.

The whole case caused an outcry, and a Canadian businessman, Edward B. Ratcliffe, went so far as to offer $1,000 to Mrs. Finkbine and any other pregnant woman in Canada or the US who wanted an abortion because she had taken the drug thalidomide. In the same year, there was an outbreak of rubella, a viral disease that also caused birth anomalies. Many people worldwide started to argue for the first time that abortion should be legalised where quality of life was an issue.

As each term at Battersea ended, I used most of my holiday period to relieve one of the Sisters in Lewes. I could not refuse my sponsors my vacation time, and besides I enjoyed going back to Sussex. Each time the train pulled into Lewes, I felt like I was coming home.

The months of college flew by, and my final ever block of nursing training was coming to an end. Exams were looming, and I was determined to do well.

'Come on, Cynthia! Take your head out of the textbooks for five minutes! Let's play some tennis; the fresh air will do you good.' I clutched the black telephone receiver in my hand, and allowed myself to be swayed by this tempting offer. It was a gorgeous spring day after all.

'OK, Peter, I'll meet you down the tennis courts in an hour.'

Peter, a police detective inspector, was my latest beau. Tall and good looking, and going places in his career, he had thick dark hair that set off the most gorgeous pair of green eyes. I liked him, and thought he had 'potential'. He was the first man I'd thought much of since Patrick.

Peter was waiting for me on the Ravenscourt tennis courts in his tennis whites, patting the balls impatiently with his wooden racquet.

'Come on, girl!' he said teasingly.

We started playing, and as I reached to return a volley during the second set, I fell heavily on my ankle. As I couldn't get up afterwards as it was too painful, Peter had to call me an ambulance. He was none too happy that I'd ruined his game of tennis. He'd been winning too!

It turned out that I'd ruptured my Achilles tendon in two places, and needed an immediate operation. Like most nurses, I was scared stiff of anaesthetics, but I was in a wonderful surgeon's hands, a Mr Hindenach at West London Hospital. I was in traction, plastered knee to ankle in an orthopaedic bed for three weeks with exams in the offing. I was cheesed off, worried that I'd be unable to sit my exams, and worse still Peter unceremoniously dumped me.

My Sister Lucille told me to look on the bright side; at least I'd seen what a selfish rat Peter was before it was too late. And, I had to admit she was right. It didn't stop me feeling sorry for myself though, as I absent-mindedly flicked through my numerous course notes.

I was anxious to get back to college so that I wouldn't miss any more course work. I was released from hospital hobbling around on a pair of crutches. Molly, Pat and Teresa were all happy to see me back again and brought me a congratulatory 'welcome back to college' coffee. They should have saved their celebrations though. On my second day back at college I fell down a flight of stairs, and was promptly sent straight back to orthopaedic ward again!

I cried with frustration and pain. Now, I definitely would not be able to sit my exams. I'd never be released from orthopaedics ward in time. However, someone must have been smiling down on me, as the powers that be at Battersea, decided to get me an ambulance to ferry me from my bed to my final oral exam. I think that they felt that because my weekly exam marks had been consistently excellent over the year, they could mark me on them. I was very glad of the Battersea Tutor's flexibility. Queen Charlottes would certainly never have done such a thing!

After nearly six years study, I was about to sit my final exam. Mum was advised to buy me a pretty dressing gown, and ensure I had nice make-up on exam day. Old-fashioned advice that was heeded, and not resented in the days before 'Women's Lib'.

The examiners ducked into the ambulance waiting outside the college and fired various questions at me. I answered as best as I could, albeit slightly doped up on painkillers.

Because of my immobile state, I missed the end of term college festivities, but the most important thing was that I was informed that I had passed my exams, and was qualified now as a Health Visitor and School Nursing Sister.

Training was finally over, there were no more exams. Now, at last I could get on with my career.

CHAPTER XV
Sussex Ups And Downs

As soon as my ankle was sufficiently healed, I went back to Sussex. During the late summer of 1962, I caught the train out of Paddington and chugged out to pastures new.

Although I was now fully qualified, I couldn't drive a car yet, having failed my test twice, so was limited in where I could be sent. I did relief work only in areas that could be adequately worked on by bicycle. I flitted between Bexhill-on-Sea, Peacehaven, Newhaven, Seaford, Pevensey Bay, Haywards Heath, Forest Row, and of course Lewes, while I waited for a suitable permanent post to come up for me.

The seaside towns had large numbers of elderly and retired folk, so most of my visits were to give baths to them. Only two of the patients on my books at Seaford were under 60! With having to lift four infirm patients in and out of their bath in any one morning, it was hard backbreaking work.

However, sometimes I assisted a patient who had hurt their own backs, not by lifting, but by becoming involved in the latest dance craze to hit the county that year. Chubby Checker's two hit singles, 'Let's Twist Again' and 'The Twist' got scores of young people twisting all over the place. The Twist was said to be the greatest thing since rock and roll. Well, my poor patient, who was only young at heart, had put their back out while twisting excessively one evening.

While I was at Newhaven, the Cuban missile crisis was at its peak, and as I had six years before during the Suez crisis of 1956, I prayed desperately that a nuclear World War III would be avoided.

The Cuban crisis began on the 14th October 1962, after an American

166

U-2 reconnaissance plane spotted Russian nuclear missiles on the Caribbean island of Cuba. The USA was within easy striking distance of Cuba, and so naturally feared the worst. President Kennedy denounced the Soviets' actions on live TV, and declared a naval blockade on Cuba, while threatening to attack the USSR if any missile were launched from Cuba against America. A huge US fleet formed an arc 500 miles from the eastern tip of Cuba, while the Soviets deployed their own ships to the island. China stepped in, backing the Russians. The world waited on tenterhooks wondering which superpower would back down first.

'The Yanks will never back down,' said nearly everybody I spoke to, 'The question is, will the Soviets back down? They're power-mad at the moment! Look at the Berlin Wall.'

'If there's a war, I'm not sure we'll win. The Commies are miles ahead of us. They got the first satellite, the first dog, and the first man in space, and hey, they even got the first rocket on the blooming moon. If there's a war we're doomed.' admitted my Newhaven housemate, Sally, as we shared some of Sister Guiness's famous Irish stew.

'Nobody can survive a nuclear war anyway. What will be left for the winners? It's pointless.' I said shuddering, once again remembering the horrific PTS film.

On the 28th October 1962, we, along with the rest of the world, could breathe again. Khrushchev had agreed to dismantle all the Russian missiles based in Cuba and ship them back to the Soviet Union.

'Thank God!' said Sally. 'That really was too close for comfort.'

'Yes, thank God.' I said, wondering when the next incident would come to cause the world to quake. It was still a very unstable peace.

The winter of 1962/63 was horrible. I had very little money, but had earmarked my last couple of pounds to come home to London on a 'flying visit' on Christmas Eve.

'Cynthia, don't come up this Christmas.' Mum advised, when I 'phoned her from a Lewes public payphone to make arrangements, 'The smog is even more awful this year. It would be dangerous for you to travel. Save your money and come up sometime in the New Year when you can enjoy it.'

I heeded her advice; The Lewisham Rail Disaster was still fresh in my memory. Smog was at its worst, and a thick layer of choking filthy fog had covered London for many days. My best friend Anne's then boyfriend, Paul, was a policeman, and he described having to manually lead traffic around Piccadilly Circus with a whistle and flag, as the fog was so thick.

London's Emergency Bed Service had admitted 235 people to hospital in a space of twenty-four hours with pneumonia and other breathing difficulties, and was on red alert status. At least one hundred Londoners had already died from health problems as a direct result of the polluted swirling mass.

I saw for myself what Mum was talking about, when Sussex was hit by the smog a few days after London. As instructed by The Ministry of Health, I warned my patients, particularly those with chest and heart problems, to stay indoors and keep all their windows and doors closed. I also demonstrated how to make do-it-yourself facemasks made from thick cotton gauze

As I cycled around in fog so bad, I could hardly see ten yards in front of me, I had my Battersea grey and maroon striped long woollen scarf wrapped around my mouth and nose. Despite these basic precautions, I still suffered from a tight chest over that period.

Although I missed being at home, I was glad I heeded Mum's advice not to travel up to London. I don't think I would have been able to get back to Sussex for some time if I had gone because of the snow.

On Boxing Day, it started to snow, and continued to snow solidly for around twenty-four hours until the snow was twelve inches deep. Being the holiday season there was little traffic, so all the roads were well and truly covered. A couple of days later there was more snow, this time accompanied by strong winds which caused snow drifts of up to four feet deep; and that was in urban areas. Cars were buried and the roads became impassable.

The winter of early 1963 was one of the coldest on record. Children had a ball, with many days off school, and seemingly endless days spent snowball fighting, skating, sledging, and building igloos and snowmen. Their creations were real works of art, many days could be spent playing in them and adding to them. Rather than two day wonders, these snow sculptures lasted most of the winter. The gigantic igloo built on one of the local village's commons didn't thaw completely until May.

It was fun for the kids, but not for me. With treacherously icy roads, a bicycle was useless in the drifts, so I was forced to walk many miles with snow up to my knees. Snow cleared from garden paths and pavements piled up in the gutter, so pavements became walled off from the road by mountains of piled up snow. The cold spell went on so long that local authorities ran out of salt to grit the roads. I'd sympathise, as I rushed past council workers, chipping away at the snow with their spades.

'Good morning, Sister. Lovely day again…' the men raised their freezing gloved hands to me as I trudged past them through the snow, ever-alert. Icicles hanging from buildings could be dangerous weapons; there were a few times that winter when I got the fright of my life, as a sharp pointed icicle fell just a few yards in front of me.

No patient ever missed a visit, although I was often very late. I'd arrive with icicles hanging from the brim of my hat, and my glass thermometers frozen in their solution within my bag. Patients relatives would attempt to wring out my overcoat and dry it before their fire, before I returned out into the snow blizzards again.

It was difficult to get water as the pipes were usually frozen. I resorted to using melted snow to boil my instruments, and to thaw my thermometers. It got so bad that the water in people's outside toilets froze, and this was a time that this was often the only toilet in the whole house.

At the height of the freeze, snow fell for thirty-six hours solid, and water froze in the main drains. As a result, I had to carry a bucket to the nearest standpipe and queue for fresh water. Luckily, when folk saw my uniform, they immediately let me get what I needed.

'Let the Nurse through! I say, let the Nurse through!' they'd cry. One kind neighbour even brought me around some water, when he knew I was in. God knows, I had little enough time to do my nursing duties, let alone to have to worry about water.

The houses where I lived were freezing, even with the fire or Rayburn lit, and ice gathered on the inside of the windows, which I'd have to scrape off each morning. It cost me a small fortune in fuel. I wore layers of thick woollen underwear, and kept my coat and gloves on all the time. Many of us nurses had nasty chilblains that winter.

Never was I gladder to see the first bloom of 1963 peep its head tentatively out, shortly after the thaws came in mid-April.

At Forest Row, there were lots of new mums. The stork had been busy in their area! I visiting the new mums and babies every day up until their fourteenth day. The new mum's houses were usually easy to spot, as they were the ones with dozens of terry towelling nappies out dancing on the washing line. One of the ladies lived in a cottage set deep within the Ashdown Forest, the inspiration for the writer of Winnie the Pooh.

The local Roman Catholic Church, 'Our Lady of the Forest' was quite stunning, and I tried to visit there whenever I had a quiet moment to myself. I felt very serene in its beautiful surroundings.

I could have kicked myself when I found out President Kennedy had paid my little church haven a visit, and I hadn't known a thing about it. On June 30th, 1963, just four days after his famous passionate 'Ich bin ein Berliner' speech given in the shadows of the Berlin wall, President Kennedy attended mass at 'Our Lady of the Forest'. Kennedy had come to Sussex to visit Prime Minister Harold Macmillan at his country home nearby.

When I later perched on one of 'Our Lady of the Forest's wooden pews, I wondered if I was sitting in the very same spot as this great man had. In Britain, The Profumo Affair scandal was at its height, forcing the resignation of The Secretary of State for War, John Profumo. I was glad that Kennedy was not such a sleazy man. (Little was I to know!)

For over a year, between 1962 and 1963, I lived like a gypsy, never staying in one place in Sussex for too long. I loved my work, but it was hard going, even when the weather was mild. No sooner had I unpacked my green trunk, than it seemed that it was time for me to move on again.

I hoped that I'd pass my driving test soon. Then nothing would stand in my way of being given my own district more or less right away. My third driving test was due, and I reported to the test centre a bag of nerves. I wondered if the driving examiner realised how much the nervous young candidate in her district nurse's uniform depended on passing her test. Thankfully, it proved to be third time lucky for me, and finally, I had a full driving license and my name could go down on East Sussex Nurses Association's list for charge of any sole district.

Two weeks after passing my test, I was asked if I wanted to take charge of the district of Bolney. Bolney was a large thriving traditional

Sussex village, and its district comprised of the nearby villages of Sayers Common, Albourne, Twineham, and Wineham.

Bolney was a pretty village coming complete with a butcher, bakers, ironmongers, Post Office, two general stores, two churches, a pub and a primary school. Bolney District was spread out over a large rural area, and would be a challenge, but one that I was more than happy to rise to. I had been trained for six years to take on such a task.

The Bolney local voluntary committee gave me the once over, at the chairman's home. The committee did a lot for the ESNA by raising funds for it by opening gardens in the Summer and other such fund-raising activities, so were given some sort of say including a 'veto' if they really did not like me. The grey-haired chairman nodded, and his elderly wife's eyes twinkled. I could see that they liked me, and I breathed a sigh of relief.

I was formally accepted to start at Bolney late Summer 1963, the same summer that the Reverend Martin Luther King gave his famous 'I have a dream' speech, The Beatles stormed the charts with 'From Me To You', and Buster Edwards and his cronies prepared for the Great Train Robbery.

As I packed up all my worldly possessions from the house that I was living in in Peacehaven, I hoped that this would be the last move my pale green trunk and I would be making for a long time. As the village bus trundled into Bolney, the wild flowers crowned their heads to greet me from their beds in the grassy lane verges.

A tabby cat dozed peacefully on the step of 1, Tythe Barne Estate, the red-bricked council house that that was to become my home. As I unlocked the door to my new home, he lazily opened his eyes, while stretching as if he had all the time in the world and blocking my entrance at the same time. I bent down to pet him, and he rubbed his head against my leg in what I took to be a traditional Bolney cat greeting. The nametag around his neck told me his name was Sammy, and that he 'officially' lived five doors away.

'Hello, Sammy! What a lovely greeting. Nice to meet you too!'

Sammy had been the first to greet me to the village. Many more would be welcoming me with open arms over the coming weeks. Sammy and I were soon to become well acquainted. He'd eat the mice and keep my feet warm, and I'd give him cuddles. Sounded like a fair enough swap to me.

~ ~ ~ ~ ~ ~ ~ ~ ~ ~ ~

I loved my time at Bolney. From 6.30am in the morning until very late, it was all go, but the warmth with which I was greeted by everyone I saw made it all worthwhile. I had little time to myself.

I could not even escape from the call of duty on my days off. The telephone rang insistently, and I'd sleepily be expected to divert the patients through to the nurse from the neighbouring district that was on duty that day in place of me. I couldn't take the 'phone off the hook, as the one day I'd tried to do this to get some much needed sleep, the BT telephone engineer had actually came to my house to ask if everything was ok, as my phone had been reported as out of order.

There was no getting away from it. Even when I popped out to get a loaf from the village shop, I was accosted by an anxious patient, who wanted to have a lengthy conversation with me about why their haemorrhoids always got worse in the cold weather. Some folk didn't seem to understand the concept of nurse having a 'day off.' Still, I wouldn't have swapped my job for the world.

East Sussex County Nursing Association by and large let me get on with it. The Area Superintendent Nursing Officer from Haywards Heath visited me on a quarterly basis, to check I was keeping my records such as my Midwives Drug Book and Register of Cases correctly, and whether I was administering my stocks of dangerous drugs in the right way. As she tucked into the roast dinner I was obliged to provide for her, the Area Superintendent Nursing Officer made meticulous notes in her neat writing and then came out with me to see some of my patients.

A pale blue Ford Anglia car, registration SPM 64, my 'company car', waited patiently for me in my garage. When East Sussex County Nursing Association had handed me over its keys on my second day in Bolney, I'd been overjoyed. My legs still ached after climbing the steep hills around Lewes on my bicycle, and I was grateful I could now finally hang up my bicycle clips.

I didn't always drive, however. I was walking back home one morning, when I saw a group of teenage girls huddled outside the local store crying. A pale-faced man stood solemnly with his grey felt hat crumpled in his hands, staring at the headline emblazoned across the newspaper board. It was 23rd November 1963.

'President Kennedy shot dead in Dallas!' the headlines screamed. It was hard to believe that the man who'd visited my favourite Church, and that had possibly even sat on the same pew as I, was dead.

'It happened late yesterday.' whispered the bystander quietly.

It was one of the few days that I allowed myself to buy a newspaper out of my limited budget. The pages were edged in black, as a sign of mourning, and most of the pages were dedicated to this shocking news. I read of JFK's last moments in the open topped car, and his beautiful wife crying, 'On no!' as she cradled her dying husband in her arms.

A few days later, I watched some flickering black and white images of the President's State funeral on one of my patient's television sets.

'That poor man!' I stared sadly at the screen, watching as a white-faced, but dignified looking, Jacqueline Kennedy, and her children, little

Caroline and three year old John Junior, paid their last respects to this great man. John Junior then heartbreakingly saluted his father's coffin.

It was the one of the only times this particular patient had beckoned me to sit down and watch a couple of minutes of TV with them. The only other time had been when I'd 'accidentally' called and interrupted my patient's enjoyment of 'Dixon of Dock Green'. I soon learned to schedule my visits around the show. It couldn't always be helped, of course!

Being a school nurse was one of my favourite parts of being on the district. At the village school, a long line of boys and girls queued up to be checked for head lice during my routine inspections every three months. Known to the teachers and parents as the nit nurse, and 'Nitty Nora' to the children, I saw each child behind a small screen, feeling through their hair for the nasty little creatures. After I checked their hair, I asked the children to 'open wide' to show me their teeth.

My check-ups weren't just about assessing hair and teeth; I assessed a child's general well being. Luckily, the children of Bolney were well cared for, and there were no signs of child abuse. In other areas, I'd sometimes spotted the telltale bruises, or lash marks on the tender flesh, and then have to take it further.

One young lad, Bob, was rather short for his age, and as this could be a sign of poor nutrition, I asked him if he ate all his dinner.

'Oh no, Miss Carstairs, I want to be a jockey just like my dad!' Bob said in horror. His dad was a jockey at a nearby Race Course. There was not a lot that I could say to that!

Several children sent me little letters and poems, and I treasured them all.

Twineham School, West Sussex. 12th January 1964

She is our District Nurse and we her patients be

She cures us when we're worse and never says fiddle de dee

Her name is Miss Carstairs

She wears a dark blue dress

For children she cares most

And always does her best

Love from Percy'

Another child wrote,

'Dear Sister Carstairs,

Do you like the Beatles? If one dies, it will rain for months.

Love Tim'

The other favourite part of my job was seeing all the babies at the monthly Infant Welfare Clinic at The Rawson Institute in Bolney. As much as I loved it, it required extra patience, as some of the babies strongly and vocally objected to being stripped naked, before being weighed on a cold iron weighing scale, despite the warming influence of a cheerful coal fire burning in the grate.

I was very lucky that some volunteers from the village such as Mrs Woodland, Mrs Philips and Mrs Seward lit these fires, and got other items ready for me at the clinic; the tins of National Dried Baby Milk that I doled out along with cod liver oil, orange juice and marmite. It made my job a lot easier.

What *didn't* make my job or energy levels easier was unthinking parents, who knocked on my door past ten at night to ask for a tin of baby milk, as they had run out. Of course, I could not deny them, although I cursed them under my breath and sternly reminded them to please get their baby milk supplies at the clinic at the proper time in future.

The Rawson Institute's annual Christmas party, held in January, had been going for years. It was great fun, and as the radio played 'The Beatles' and 'Gerry and the Pacemakers' latest singles, babies jiggled and arm-jived on their mother's laps. The night before the 1964 Christmas party, I'd been up making cakes and jellies for thirty-four invited guests, until way past midnight. All the baking ingredients had to be provided at my own expense. I wouldn't have grudged it, except I could hardly afford to feed myself, let alone thirty-four other mouths.

I lived off baked beans, cracked eggs, sardines on toast and other such cheap food, and loans from Mum until the end of month. I hardly lived a frivolous lifestyle. It was just after paying the rent and bills, there was very little left to live on.

Letters from Mum suggested I make a little extra money by selling homemade blackberry and apple jam. That autumn, I'd used a precious day off to go to a pretty country lane to fill my basket with juicy Sussex berries. I then made what seemed like dozens of pots of jam, which I decorated with cheerful gingham cloth lids. I made a few shillings from my efforts, which quickly went straight back out to pay the chimney sweep to unblock the chimney.

Sometimes one of the local farmers generously gave me some of their homemade produce, or a basketful of organic vegetables. Once I was even given a whole plucked pheasant by a patient. As this patient was a bit of character, having a reputation, I heard later, as a bit of a poacher, the pheasant probably came from dubious sources, but I gratefully received his gift none the less.

'Thanks, Mr Cox.' I smiled.

'And 'ere's a bottle of home brew for yer' nurse, it ain't 'arf good nurse, it'll do yer' good.' His brown eyes twinkled mischievously.

'Thanks again, Mr Cox!'

As I didn't drink, I gave the bottle to my mum, who declared it was the best home brew she'd ever tasted. Looking back on it, I should have drunk it. On my days off when patients rang incessantly from 6am until 9pm, and fathers knocked on the door at 10pm for a tin of baby milk, I'm sure it would have 'done me good'.

CHAPTER XVI

'Don't forget to put the Kettle on'

'Sister, I'm so sorry to call you out at this unearthly hour, but it's my wife. She's started and the pains are coming now every ten minutes. Please hurry.'

Before the anxious father-to-be said anymore a rush of adrenaline woke me up. It was finally happening! My first Bolney baby was about to be born! Clutching the black Bakelite telephone by my bed, I replied,

'Yes, of course, Mr Harvey, I'll come right away.' I paused for a moment: the Harvey's house was located out 'in the sticks' and there were no streetlights. 'Please switch on all the house lights at the front for me, and draw back the curtains, so I can find my way up the lane. I know where you are but this will help me to get you quicker.' Then jokingly I added, 'Don't forget to put the kettle on'.

I didn't want the hot water for a cup of tea. The water was needed to boil up my midwifery instruments and bowls. However, tea would not be unwelcome to the labouring patient and her midwife.

Ready for a speedy getaway, only three hours before this nocturnal telephone call, I had laid out my cornflower blue short-sleeved uniform dress with its detachable semi-stiff white collar and cuffs, and carefully placed my black SRN's belt and polished black leather shoes close to hand. My hat, coat and white gloves were waiting for me in the hallway, hanging up on the dark wooden coat-stand.

Quickly dressing, and then checking my reflection carefully in the mirror, I adjusted my precious Queen's Nurses Bronze Medal on its two-colour blue cord, so that it hung exactly two inches from my collar.

It was now 1964, and I was twenty-six years old.

'Bye, Sammy!' I called to my new furry best-friend, 'keep my bed warm for me!'

I was really tired, and there was nothing more that I wanted than to go back to bed. The day before had been an exceptionally busy day, and I had hoped for a restful night's sleep. The Infant Welfare Clinic earlier had been hectic, much as I expected. The effects of the post-war baby boom were all around me giggling, sneezing or wailing. After the last baby had been weighed and checked, I'd then had to rush out to one of my cancer patients in neighbouring Twineham.

Mrs Smith was a thirty-eight year old mother in the last stages of terminal breast cancer. She had rapidly deteriorated over the past few days and I needed to give her morphine injections every four hours.

Knowing her end was close, Mrs Smith refused to go back into hospital, preferring to be surrounded by her husband and toddler son, Ben, and Rex, her black Labrador dog, who watched my every move suspiciously.

'I've got my eye on you, Nurse!' Rex seemed to hint, 'Just you make sure you get that jab right!'

It was my privileged duty to carry out the family's request to enable Mrs Smith to live her last days in her home, but it meant no early nights for me, as at 10pm each night I had to attend to her.

And so I had earlier that night. After giving Mrs Smith her Morphine injection to ease her pain and help her to sleep, I gave her a quick wash, put a comb through her hair, and changed her bed sheets.

'Call me if you need anything. *Anytime.*' I'd insisted to her grey-faced husband, as he showed me to the front door. The reassurance that I, or another Nursing sister would return at any time if called, was just part of the total nursing care a Queen's Nursing Sister was expected to provide. Mr Smith clung desperately to his young son, Ben, as much to comfort himself as to comfort his son. I knew Mr Smith hadn't accepted his wife was dying yet. There was still hope there; hope and desperation in his eyes.

'Remember, call me.' I said.

I left the Smiths at 10.30pm as a cancer care nurse, and now just five hours later, my role was changing as I was called upon by the Harvey family to use my training and skills as a State Certified Midwife.

My Midwives' Register of Cases, which by law I had to keep for the rest of my life, noted that most of the little ones I delivered, chose, for reasons best known to themselves, to make their entrance into the world in the middle of the night. The Harvey's child was proving no exception to this rule.

I hurried out into the frosty night, clutching the heavy gas and air machine in one hand and my two midwifery bags in the other. I was glad that although it was cold, there was no snow on the ground. Thank goodness this winter wasn't like last year's, I thought. I certainly didn't feel like trudging five miles in the snowdrifts to the Harvey's farm tonight.

I looked at my Timex nurse's watch with a second hand that had lasted me all the way from the beginning of my Nursing adventure at Preliminary Training School. It was just gone 3.30am in the morning, and I'd be at the Harvey's farm in less than twenty minutes.

I was to be in sole charge of this delivery and I knew that both the lives of the mother and her unborn child depended on my skills. It was a solemn responsibility, but six year's grind had prepared me and given me confidence for this task. Dr Madison, the Harvey's GP, came out to assist only if I called him for medical assistance. I was left by the East Sussex County Nursing Association to 'get on with it.' I determined I would do this all by myself. This labour would go fine. It had to!

Following the tradition passed on by Sister Holland and the other Queenies, who had worked this district before me, I quickly picked up a piece of white chalk and scribbled on a small '12 x 12' blackboard, 'Cherry Tree Farm, phone 206'. I then placed the board in full view on the window ledge by my back door. Now other patients needing me would know where I was, and how to contact me. As a back-up, all my midwifery patients had 'just in case,' the telephone number of Sisters Gordon-Watson & Pembleton, of the neighbouring district of Hurstpierpoint, known as 'Hurst' to the locals.

I shivered as the cold night air hit me, pulling my navy gabardine coat tight to myself, as I made my way to unlock my unlit garage. I nearly jumped out of my skin when an owl loudly hooted from the nearby trees.

'Don't be so silly, Cynthia,' I scolded myself. I wasn't sure why I felt so nervous. I always felt a flurry of excitement about a baby being born, but I didn't normally feel as anxious as this. Taking a deep breath, I tried to maintain my composure as I pulled myself together. Yes, the eyes of the village were upon me, but I would not let them down. After all, I hadn't done yet, had I?

Having a car made things so much easier, and was a valuable time saver. I had no fear of being alone on the dark country lanes at this time of the morning. It didn't even enter my head that I was a potential target as I was carrying a dangerously addictive drug Pethilorfan. Although there was some drug-misuse, it was small and relatively manageable, contained in the major urban areas. I was still a few years away from the Hippie Culture, and the explosion of drug taking for recreational use. Brighton had not yet become the anything goes Bohemian pleasure centre it would later be noted for.

I'd got to know the little winding roads that led out to the surrounding villages well in the few months I'd been at Bolney. As I drove along the Village High Street, turning onto the A23 heading for 'Cherry Tree Farm', I was pumped with adrenaline, my mind on the labouring Mrs Harvey.

'It should go alright.' I thought, 'She's healthy and had two easy labours before.' Of course, there were no guarantees, and I could not rely on my rule of thumb to be the law.

I had got to know Mrs Harvey and the rest of her family during her antenatal period. Choosing to visit Cherry Tree Farm after school time, had enabled me to get to meet the two Harvey's two daughters, Sally and Emily, as well as enabling me to catch the anxious father-to-be in-between milking his herd of cows. It was important that the whole family got involved with the new baby.

'Nurse, please can you bring us a brother?' asked Sally, looking at me pleadingly from beneath her golden fringe, as she clutching her beloved rag doll to herself. 'I will really help out Mummy with him…' Sally at aged six, the eldest, and therefore the spokeswoman of the sisters, continued to chatter about her brother, her green eyes shining with enthusiasm. 'We want a brother don't we, Emily?'

'Yes!' Emily, age four, bent down and peered suspiciously into my black bag. Few children knew about 'the birds and bees' then, and a common myth was that baby popped out of Sister's black bag.

'I'll see what I can do, girls.' I winked at their mum. What did Mrs Harvey have curled up inside her snug and warm? No one knew, it was pure guesswork. In 1964, apart from the plentiful old wives tales and the pendulum, there were no special tools to determine the unborn baby's sex, but then that was half the fun!

'Any names in mind yet?' I had asked the still expanding, waddling and breathless Mrs Harvey just three days before.

'Paul after Paul McCartney for a boy, and Jacqueline after the late American President's wife for a girl. As long as the baby's alright we don't really mind, Nurse, but I'd be so grateful for a little boy this time. We do reckon it's a boy though, because of the amount the baby's been kicking!'

'You're having a little footballer then!' I said jokily, 'And you are carrying high. A midwife I worked with at Queen Charlotte's Hospital swore that meant you'll have a boy.'

'We'll see,' smiled Mrs Harvey. I noted that most of the tiny knitted cardigans and baby booties Mrs Harvey had been working on, whenever I'd seen her, had been of a pale blue colour. I hoped she wouldn't be disappointed.

As I came down the bumpy country lane that led off the A23, it was easy to spot Cherry Tree Farm from half a mile away, with all its lights ablaze. An anxious Mr Harvey quickly opened the front door when I was still only halfway down the leaf strewn path, and a draught of warm air greeted me as I entered the cosy farmhouse.

'Thank you for coming so quickly, Sister, we're sorry to get you out of your bed on a night like this.' Mr Harvey gabbled apologetically. 'I'll make you a nice cup of tea, the kettle's not long boiled.'

He led me upstairs to his anxious panting wife, who was relieved to see me. On the way up, I brushed past their four-year old daughter, Emily, whose eyes were nearly popping out of her head.

'Go back to bed!' Mr Harvey ordered, and there was a light scampering of two pairs of little feet running down the landing with giggles and whispers. As I approached Mrs Harvey's bed, I could immediately see she was in an advanced stage of labour.

'Don't worry about the tea for now, Mr Harvey, please boil these instruments for ten minutes for me.' I handed him over several stainless steel bowls and instruments. It was far better to keep him occupied elsewhere, and not have him under my feet, as I checked exactly how far advanced in labour his wife was.

I took off my hat and coat and folded it into a neat pile. I carefully placed it on newspaper covering the Bakelite table. This ritual was to prevent damage to furniture, and crucially to stop household fleas jumping on my clothes. The Harvey's were a clean family but it was important to keep up my training – one never knew!

There were already some items waiting for me at the Harvey's in a large brown cardboard box that I had taken around only three weeks earlier. It was labelled 'not to open until needed'. Provided by East Sussex County Council, it was full of maternity pads, cotton wool, baby's cord powder, and a large brown paper plastic backed sheet to protect the new mum's mattress from blood and other mess.

I had instructed the family to cover the expectant mother's bed mattress with clean newspapers, and then cover this layer of newspapers with the brown waterproof cover in case labour started suddenly with early rupture of the membranes (the waters breaking). The Harvey family had also been instructed to collect a pile of newspapers for me to use to protect their furniture and carpets.

I dressed so that no germs could pass from me to Mum and baby, putting on a long white gown over my uniform, and ensuring that I covered every scrap of my hair with a clean, triangular piece of cotton made into a cap.

As I examined Mrs Harvey, I made note of my findings, such as the pulse rate, the dilation of the cervix, and the timing of the contractions with my blue parker fountain pen, given me for my 21st birthday by Patrick.

Luckily, baby Harvey was the 'right way around', lying headfirst. I listened to baby's heartbeat using a small metal trumpet shaped stethoscope. The heartbeat needed to be recorded because any change in the rhythm indicated distress and would require me to call for medical aid to get the baby delivered as quickly as possible, possibly by caesarean section operation.

There was an excellent Obstetric Flying Squad based at Brighton that I could call out if necessary. It was reassuring to have this back-up unit standing by, complete with saline, bottles of blood, warmed blankets and consultant obstetrician and senior midwife. They could be with me in minutes. I later did have to make use of this service for one patient, a Mrs Donald, who suddenly lost a lot of blood and needed an emergency transfusion to save her life.

My trusty gas and air machine hardly seemed to be touching Mrs Harvey's pain.

'Would you like an injection of Pethilorfan to help the contractions?' I asked Mrs Harvey. (Yes, of course, it is pain, but we midwives were taught to call this pain contractions!)

'What do you think, Sister?' I had to use my judgement wisely. Pethilorfan can harm the baby given too near the birth.

'It will help you a lot'. I hastened to drawn up the valuable drug in its correct dose in a freshly sterilised glass hypodermic syringe, and administered it to Mrs Harvey.

Mr Harvey waited tentatively at the bedroom door, not sure if he was allowed to come in or not. I motioned to him to enter and then quickly covered the bedside table with newspapers. The rest of the newly boiled equipment handed over helpfully by Mr Harvey, was neatly laid out with gloved hands and covered over with a sterile cotton cloth.

Amongst the instruments ready at my side, were Spencer Wells artery forceps to clamp the baby's umbilical cord, cord ligatures and scissors. Another glass hypodermic syringe was on standby, which would be later filled with the drug Ergometrine, routinely used to help the mother's uterus contract to its pre-pregnancy size and to help prevent further bleeding.

'You're nearly fully dilated. Baby won't be too much longer…and it will soon be time to push. I think we all deserve that brew now, eh, Mr Harvey?'

Mr Harvey arrived back upstairs laden down with a tea tray, on which was neatly laid out the family's best china on a pretty lace cloth. Although he looked somewhat heated and flustered (not used to having to make the tea, no doubt) it was a lovely cup of tea nonetheless.

The Pethilorfan injection worked quickly, soothing the labouring mother a little, and I enjoyed a glorious cup of tea, all the while keeping a careful eye on mum and baby's pulse rates. I could not relax for one second – so many complications could still occur. At every moment, I had to be fully alert, as one mistake could prove fatal. I let Mr Harvey listen to his baby's heartbeat on my stethoscope. 'Patter, patter…' to the tune of around one hundred and twenty beats a minute. What a lovely sound!

Was it a boy or girl? Possibly, albeit rarely, there were two little bundles of joy curled up inside, when only one was expected! That had happened to my friend, Carla, on her 'beat' in Hastings. A Simpson's trained midwife, and therefore one of the best midwives in the country, it proved that in the days before ultra-sound, these sort of mistakes could still happen.

'It's time to push, Mrs Harvey. Doctor Madison will come out if we need him, but we can manage this between ourselves, don't you agree? Besides you are an old hand at this, you've done this twice before!' I reassured the anxious mum with a little chuckle.

I asked Mr Harvey if he wanted to stay to watch the arrival.

Midwifery was not yet at a point where a midwife would allow a father to cut the umbilical cord, but at least they could watch during home births. Men had been known to faint on such occasions; I vividly remembered one new father in Walthamstow keeling over at the sight of all the blood, so I had to be careful to avoid having a third patient at Cherry Tree Farm, a collapsed Mr Harvey, to look after as well.

Getting ready for the immanent arrival, I placed a cotton facemask over my face to prevent droplet infection, and covered my hands in sterile rubber gloves.

The pushing phase was over in a matter of minutes. Very quickly, Mr Harvey has a glimpse of the final forceful contraction of the uterine muscles that forced out a warm slippery baby boy into my guiding hands. Paul Harvey had finally made his entrance to the world. It was 5.45am.

The look of worry on Mr Harvey's weatherworn face was now replaced by a delighted grin.

'Congratulation, it's a boy! I'm so pleased you got what you wanted.' I smiled. And I had got what I had wanted, a trouble-free labour.

I gently turned Paul upside down to allow his mouth to drain of any fluids that had collected there, before quickly wiping his mouth with cotton wool that had been sterilised by being baked in the oven in an Oxo tin. As he hung upside down, Paul took his first breath, and the world heard his voice for the first time.

'Hello, Paul, what you singing for us?' asked his Beatle-mad dad.

I cleaned Paul up a little more, wiping his eyes and ears free of mucus. He looked up at me sleepily, rather surprised by the all the light and new noises. I cut the umbilical cord and tied it off, using two ligatures in case one should slip. Then Paul was wrapped in a clean towel that had been warming over a Boots's hot rubber water bottle, and handed over to Mum for his first cuddle. Mrs Harvey smiled as her new son was placed in her arms. Mr Harvey looked on proudly, before giving his exhausted wife a big kiss.

'Thank you, Sister' they both nodded at me.

'You're welcome!' I was nearly as thrilled as they were. I felt like crying, I felt like singing. All the hard work I'd gone through during six years training was worth this one moment. All I wanted to do was relish the moment and goggle at the new baby, but my work was not yet finished.

I couldn't relax yet, as my mind was rapidly working through the process of the third stage of labour. I needed to be vigilant, as haemorrhage was a killer in these latter stages.

Ensuring that the mothers' afterbirth was complete, I wrapped it up together with the soiled swabs and newspapers and quickly tucked the grisly package into the family's burning Rayburn. Bleeding from Mrs Harvey's uterus was minimal, but I injected the routine Ergometrine anyway, whilst checking her already naturally contracting uterus.

'It's time for your first bath now, Paul!' I said, splashing the warm bath water lathered with Johnson's baby soap around the family's washing up bowl. After I gave him a quick dip, I gently patted Paul dry with a warm towel, and checked that the new baby had all his little fingers and toes and appeared 'normal'. I weighed Paul on the set of scales I carried around with me, and recorded his weight in my register, 7lbs 7oz.

Luckily, Paul's cord stump had stopped bleeding, and he was now contentedly blinking at his parents, while they cooed delightedly at him. His cord stump was cleaned and dressed with sterile dressings and special cord powder and he was ready to be dressed in all his finery in a tiny cherub fine wool vest and cotton gown with back ties. An Ashton's Zorbit soft cotton terry towelling napkin was put in place, held securely without the use of safety pins.

It was time to give the sweaty Mother a refreshing blanket bath. Paul was placed in his father's arms, as I got Mrs Harvey bathed. Mr Harvey suddenly looked rather worried. He obviously wasn't used to being left to hold the baby.

After removing the plastic sheets and newspapers from the bed, and making the bed up clean and fresh, I ensured Mrs Harvey was propped up comfortably in bed. With brushed teeth, and combed hair, and wearing a clean nightie and a fresh maternity pad, Mrs Harvey almost felt human again. Mrs Harvey, an old hand, needed no guidance or reassurance to lift her new son to her breast for his first meal.

The sound of whispering was heard outside the slightly ajar bedroom door. 'You have a little brother, Paul.' I heard Mr Harvey tell the girls,

'Yes!' excited little voices squealed with glee, 'We knew Sister Carstairs wouldn't let us down!'

All my instruments and bowls needed re-sterilised by boiling on the Rayburn, before being packed away. Mr Harvey had been quite amused by my so called 'District Nurse's paper bag' made in origami fashion by a large sheet of newspaper, and placed on the floor to collect up all my bits as I packed away.

'A cup of tea all round, please, Mr Harvey' I grinned, finally taking a seat to start making the detailed nursing notes necessary both for my register and for Doctor Madison to read on his visit later. I left the brown manila envelope labelled 'nursing notes' on the mantle-piece for the Doctor and Relief Nursing Sisters to see. In turn, the doctor would write notes inside for me to read, and thereby we'd exchange ideas and make requests of each other without actually talking to each other.

As I sipped on my tea, I finished writing my notes and watched the excited sisters peeping at their lovely new baby brother. Paul was now sleeping peacefully on his mum's breast, swathed up warm and protectively in a Zorbit blanket.

'Can I phone Doctor Madison before I go?' I enquired. At least 7.30am was now a reasonable hour to call the doctor to inform him that he now had a new patient on his books. I would be back in an hour or two anyway. It was law for the delivering midwife to return to the new mother within four hours after the birth however busy, or tired she felt, or whatever the hour of day or night.

'Look after Mummy and Paul, won't you Sally and Emily?' I called, as I headed out the front door.

I finally left Cherry Tree farm at 7.40am. Mr Harvey and the girls waved me off, full of thanks and praise for my service. A wave of exhaustion hit me as soon as I started up the car ignition, and I struggled to keep my eyes open. Even though it was cold, I cranked down the car window, so the fresh air would keep me alert. There'd just be time for a cup of coffee and a bowl of cornflakes before I had to head out again. I'd get a 'second wind' soon enough, I always did. I knew that from experience after having skipped many a night's sleep. Dear old Sammy had been keeping my bed warm for nothing.

Despite my tiredness and aching back, as I drove home through the gorgeous little villages in my little blue Ford Anglia, I felt very privileged. What a rewarding job I had, and what a lot I had to be grateful for. A safe delivery and a boy just as 'ordered' – it couldn't have worked out better.

When I'd let Patrick go, some people had said to me that I'd left the love of my love for nursing. Now I knew they were wrong; *nursing* was the love of my life.

Epilogue
2004

Cynthia' spirit did not give in, however her back did.

In late 1964, her weak back forced her to leave the district and people she had grown to love, and she reluctantly returned to London. Cynthia worked as a School Nurse & Health Visitor in South London throughout the 1960s.

She eventually married in 1969, giving birth to twins a year later.

Cynthia is now retired from nursing, and lives in Sussex with her cat Edward, within a stone's throw of her beloved South Downs. She writes and lectures on nursing history.

The children and even the grandchildren of the babies Cynthia delivered are now running around in the school playgrounds, and as she watches the children at play, Cynthia says,

'How privileged I am to have worked in one of the most noble of professions.'

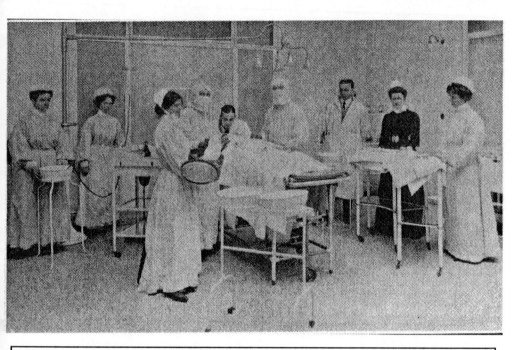